T0259246

Lower Extremity Complex Trauma and Complications

Editor

JOHN J. STAPLETON

CLINICS IN PODIATRIC MEDICINE AND SURGERY

www.podiatric.theclinics.com

Consulting Editor
THOMAS ZGONIS

October 2014 • Volume 31 • Number 4

ELSEVIER

1600 John F. Kennedy Boulevard ● Suite 1800 ● Philadelphia, Pennsylvania, 19103-2899

http://www.theclinics.com

CLINICS IN PODIATRIC MEDICINE AND SURGERY Volume 31, Number 4
October 2014 ISSN 0891-8422, ISBN-13: 978-0-323-32630-8

Editor: Jennifer Flynn-Briggs
Developmental Editor: Casey Jackson

Clinics in Podiatric Medicine and Surgery (ISSN 0891-8422) is published quarterly by Elsevier Inc., 360 Park Avenue South, New York, NY 10010-1710. Months of issue are January, April, July, and October. Business and Editorial Offices: 1600 John F. Kennedy Blvd., Ste. 1800, Philadelphia, PA 19103-2899. Customer Service Office: 3251 Riverport Lane, Maryland Heights, MO 63043. Periodicals postage paid at New York, NY and additional mailing offices. Subscription prices are $305.00 per year for US individuals, $450.00 per year for US institutions, $155.00 per year for US students and residents, $370.00 per year for Canadian individuals, $544.00 for Canadian institutions, $435.00 for international individuals, $544.00 per year for international institutions and $220.00 per year for Canadian and foreign students/residents. To receive student/resident rate, orders must be accompanied by name of affiliated institution, date of term, and the *signature* of program/residency coordinator on institution letterhead. Orders will be billed at individual rate until proof of status is received. Foreign air speed delivery is included in all *Clinics* subscription prices. All prices are subject to change without notice. POSTMASTER: Send address changes to *Clinics in Podiatric Medicine and Surgery*, Elsevier Health Sciences Division, Subscription Customer Service, 3251 Riverport Lane, Maryland Heights, MO 63043. **Customer Service: 1-800-654-2452 (US). From outside of the US, call 314-447-8871. Fax: 314-447-8029. E-mail: JournalsCustomerService-usa@elsevier.com (for print support); JournalsOnlineSupport-usa@elsevier. com (for online support).**

Reprints. For copies of 100 or more of articles in this publication, please contact the Commercial Reprints Department, Elsevier Inc., 360 Park Avenue South, New York, NY 10010-1710. Tel.: 212-633-3874; Fax: 212-633-3820; E-mail: reprints@elsevier.com.

Clinics in Podiatric Medicine and Surgery is covered in *MEDLINE/PubMed (Index Medicus)* and *EMBASE/Excerpta Medica*.

Contributors

CONSULTING EDITOR

THOMAS ZGONIS, DPM, FACFAS
Associate Professor, Externship and Fellowship Director in Reconstructive Foot and Ankle Surgery, Division of Podiatric Medicine and Surgery, Department of Orthopaedic Surgery, University of Texas Health Science Center at San Antonio, San Antonio, Texas

EDITOR

JOHN J. STAPLETON, DPM, FACFAS
Associate, Foot and Ankle Surgery, VSAS Orthopaedics, Chief of Podiatric Surgery, Lehigh Valley Hospital, Allentown, Pennsylvania; Clinical Assistant Professor of Surgery, Penn State College of Medicine, Hershey, Pennsylvania

AUTHORS

PATRICK BURNS, DPM
Assistant Professor, University of Pittsburgh Medical Center Mercy Hospital, Comprehensive Foot and Ankle Center, Pittsburgh, Pennsylvania

YURY BYKOV, MD
Orthopaedic Trauma Surgeon, Orthopaedic Surgery, VSAS Orthopaedics, Lehigh Valley Hospital, Allentown, Pennsylvania

LAWRENCE A. DiDOMENICO, DPM, FACFAS
Ankle and Foot Care Centers, Youngstown, Ohio; Adjunct Professor, Director of Reconstructive Rearfoot and Ankle Surgical Fellowship, Kent State University College of Podiatric Medicine, Independence, Ohio; Teaching staff, Heritage Valley Health System, Beaver, Pennsylvania

GEOFFREY G. HALLOCK, MD
Division of Plastic Surgery, Sacred Heart Hospital and Lehigh Valley Hospital, Allentown, Pennsylvania; St Luke's Hospital, Bethlehem, Pennsylvania

PETE HIGHLANDER, DPM, MS
PGY-3 UPMC, Podiatric Medicine and Surgery Residency, University of Pittsburgh Medical Center Mercy Hospital, Comprehensive Foot and Ankle Center, Pittsburgh, Pennsylvania

KALLIOPI LAMPROPOULOU-ADAMIDOU, MD, MSc
3rd Department of Orthopaedics and Traumatology, KAT Hospital, Kifisia, Athens, Greece

SPIROS G. PNEUMATICOS, MD, PhD
3rd Department of Orthopaedics and Traumatology, KAT Hospital, Kifisia, Athens, Greece

VASILIOS D. POLYZOIS, MD, PhD
3rd Department of Orthopaedics and Traumatology, KAT Hospital, Kifisia, Athens, Greece

CRYSTAL L. RAMANUJAM, DPM, MSc
Assistant Professor/Clinical, Division of Podiatric Medicine and Surgery, Department of Orthopaedic Surgery, University of Texas Health Science Center at San Antonio, San Antonio, Texas

SCOTT E. SEXTON, MD
Director of Orthopaedic Trauma, Department of Surgery, Lehigh Valley Hospital, VSAS Orthopaedics, Allentown, Pennsylvania

ANDREW B. SHINABARGER, DPM, MS
Legacy Medical Group - Foot and Ankle, Portland, Oregan

JOHN J. STAPLETON, DPM, FACFAS
Associate, Foot and Ankle Surgery, VSAS Orthopaedics, Chief of Podiatric Surgery, Lehigh Valley Hospital, Allentown, Pennsylvania; Clinical Assistant Professor of Surgery, Penn State College of Medicine, Hershey, Pennsylvania

IOANNIS P. STATHOPOULOS, MD, MSc
3rd Department of Orthopaedics and Traumatology, KAT Hospital, Kifisia, Athens, Greece

ZACHARY M. THOMAS, DPM
Ankle and Foot Care Centers, Youngstown, Ohio; Heritage Valley Health System, Beaver, Pennsylvania

ELIAS S. VASILIADIS, MD, PhD
3rd Department of Orthopaedics and Traumatology, KAT Hospital, Kifisia, Athens, Greece

JOHN VLAMIS, MD, PhD
3rd Department of Orthopaedics and Traumatology, KAT Hospital, Kifisia, Athens, Greece

GEORGE F. WALLACE, DPM, MBA
Director, Podiatry Service; Medical Director, University Hospital, Newark, New Jersey

THOMAS ZGONIS, DPM, FACFAS
Associate Professor, Externship and Fellowship Director in Reconstructive Foot and Ankle Surgery, Division of Podiatric Medicine and Surgery, Department of Orthopaedic Surgery, University of Texas Health Science Center at San Antonio, San Antonio, Texas

Contents

Open fractures of the lower extremity cover a wide gamut of injuries ranging from the mangled, pulseless leg necessitating amputation to the more innocuous pinhole open wounds associated with simple fracture patterns. Prompt diagnosis and appropriate care can make a dramatic difference in decreasing complication rates and improving ultimate outcomes. Principles of management of open fractures have been created with the main goal of decreasing infection rates, while providing for stabilization of the bone and soft tissue injury.

One of the most devastating foot and/or ankle complications in the diabetic population with peripheral neuropathy is the presence of Charcot neuroarthropathy (CN). In recent years, diabetic limb salvage has been attempted more frequently as opposed to major lower extremity amputation for CN of the foot and ankle with ulceration and/or deep infection. Treatment strategies for osteomyelitis in the diabetic population have evolved. This article reviews some of the most common surgical strategies recommended for the diabetic patient with CN of the foot and/or ankle and concomitant osteomyelitis.

Treatment of midfoot injuries is surgical or nonsurgical, depending on the injury, the location, and the extent of the injury. Minor injuries usually heal with casting or bracing, whereas more unstable injuries typically need surgery for stability. Whether the injury is in a weight-bearing portion of the foot is also a consideration for surgery. The importance of treating midfoot injuries adequately is shown in how the midfoot is needed for function with weight bearing and its relationship between the front and the back of the foot. It is also important to ensure that the patient is able to ambulate with a reasonably normal gait.

CLINICS IN PODIATRIC MEDICINE AND SURGERY

NOW AVAILABLE FOR YOUR iPhone and iPad

Foreword

Lower Extremity Trauma and Complications

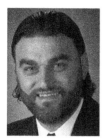

Thomas Zgonis, DPM, FACFAS
Consulting Editor

This issue of *Clinics in Podiatric Medicine and Surgery* focuses on the surgical management of lower extremity trauma and its complications. Various topics from tibial plafond fractures to midfoot crush injuries and rehabilitation are well covered by the experienced authors and invited guest editor, Dr John J. Stapleton. These highly complex injuries are best managed in trauma centers where trauma protocols are well established in dealing with limb-threatening and/or life-threatening injuries. Complex lower extremity injuries are often associated with multiple body injuries that may need to be addressed in an urgent/emergent basis.

Surgical experience and training are paramount in dealing with the complex foot and ankle trauma, including knowledge in the management of major osseous and soft tissue defects. In this issue, the guest editor and the invited authors have done an excellent job in addressing some of the most common complex lower extremity injuries that can be used as a great guidance to our readers. Finally, I am thankful to all of your continuous efforts and contributions to the *Clinics in Podiatric Medicine and Surgery*.

Thomas Zgonis, DPM, FACFAS
Division of Podiatric Medicine and Surgery
Department of Orthopaedic Surgery
University of Texas Health Science Center at San Antonio
7703 Floyd Curl Drive MSC 7776
San Antonio, TX 78229, USA

E-mail address:
zgonis@uthscsa.edu

Clin Podiatr Med Surg 31 (2014) xiii
http://dx.doi.org/10.1016/j.cpm.2014.07.002
0891-8422/14/$ – see front matter © 2014 Elsevier Inc. All rights reserved.
podiatric.theclinics.com

Preface

Lower Extremity Complex Trauma and Complications

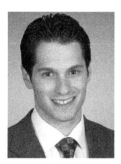

John J. Stapleton, DPM, FACFAS
Editor

I am honored to serve as a guest editor in this issue of *Clinics in Podiatric Medicine and Surgery* that is dedicated to the management of complex foot and ankle trauma. I am also thankful to the invited authors who are mostly actively practicing at Level 1 trauma facilities to devote their time and share the most current strategies for the management of lower extremity injuries. Providing optimal patient care from the initial treatment to rehabilitation is essential in the patient's successful outcome in every trauma protocol.

The care of complex foot and ankle trauma is best handled by an interdisciplinary surgical team that most frequently encounters patients with isolated or multilevel trauma injuries. High-energy foot and ankle trauma is often associated with multiple skeletal and/or life-threatening injuries. For these reasons, it is essential that the foot and ankle surgeon work efficiently and effectively in an interdisciplinary team model, including but not limited to orthopedic trauma, general surgery trauma, and plastic reconstructive services. In addition, surgical expertise with soft tissue coverage of open fractures or large open wounds is paramount in the management of the mangled lower extremity.

Finally, I would like to thank my family for all of their support as well as all of the authors for their time and contributions. I hope you enjoy reading this issue and come away with learning new strategies to improve the care of the patient with complex lower extremity trauma.

John J. Stapleton, DPM, FACFAS
Foot and Ankle Surgery
VSAS Orthopaedics
Allentown, PA, USA

E-mail address:
jostaple@hotmail.com

Clin Podiatr Med Surg 31 (2014) xv
http://dx.doi.org/10.1016/j.cpm.2014.07.001
0891-8422/14/$ – see front matter © 2014 Published by Elsevier Inc.

Open Fractures of the Foot and Ankle

Scott E. Sexton, MD

KEYWORDS

- Open fractures • Lower extremity • Foot

KEY POINTS

- Open fractures of the lower extremity cover a wide gamut of injuries ranging from the mangled, pulseless leg necessitating amputation to the more innocuous pinhole open wounds associated with simple fracture patterns.
- Prompt diagnosis and appropriate care can make a dramatic difference in decreasing complication rates and improving ultimate outcomes.
- Principles of management of open fractures have been created with the main goal of decreasing infection rates, while providing for stabilization of the bone and soft tissue injury.

INTRODUCTION

Open fractures of the lower extremity cover a wide gamut of injuries ranging from the mangled, pulseless leg necessitating amputation to the more innocuous pinhole open wounds associated with simple fracture patterns. Prompt diagnosis and appropriate care can make a dramatic difference in decreasing complication rates and improving ultimate outcomes. In general, open fractures result from high-energy injuries, resulting in varying degrees of soft tissue and skeletal damage. There is often significant periosteal stripping at the fracture site and compromised vascularity. The open wound allows communication between the outside environment and the fractured bone, and resultant hematoma, allowing for contamination of the wound with microorganisms. These factors result in a much greater risk of infection in open fractures than closed fractures.

Principles of management of open fractures have been created with the main goal of decreasing infection rates, while providing for stabilization of the bone and soft tissue injury. The current treatment of open fractures is evolving. Many long-standing guidelines based on little to no scientific evidence have been challenged including the golden 6-hour rule to debridement. This review addresses generalized principles

Disclosure: None.
Department of Surgery, Lehigh Valley Hospital, VSAS Orthopaedics, 1250 South Cedar Crest Boulevard, Allentown, PA 18103, USA
E-mail address: bbsloane2@excite.com

and management strategies for open fractures as well as looks specifically at certain common injuries in the foot and ankle region.

CLASSIFICATION OF OPEN FRACTURES

Classification systems are beneficial when they are simple, can guide treatment, and predict outcome. Open fractures are most often classified using the system outlined by Gustilo and Anderson.[1] A thorough analysis of the patient with an open fracture must be performed before assigning a score. Factors that must be considered include the mechanism of injury, degree of soft tissue damage, fracture characteristics, and degree of contamination. An initial score can be assigned on presentation; however, the most accurate and reliable score cannot be determined until after surgical debridement.

Type I fractures have puncture wounds (<1 cm), with simple fracture patterns, little soft tissue damage, and minimal contamination.

Type II fractures have larger wounds (1–10 cm), with moderate soft tissue damage. Fracture patterns are generally simple with mild comminution, and bone coverage is adequate.

Type III fractures involve extensive soft tissue damage and fractures with segmental patterns and extensive comminution. Heavy contamination can also be present. Type III fractures are subclassified into A, B, and C groups.

Group A: marked by the presence of extensive soft tissue damage with adequate bone coverage

Group B: marked by stripping of periosteum and exposed bone; bone coverage is not adequate

Group C: marked by the presence of vascular injury necessitating repair.

This scoring system remains the most widely taught and used because it meets the goals of being simple, guiding treatment, and predicting outcome, especially risk for complications. In general, the higher the score, the greater the degree of both soft tissue and bony injury and the greater the risk of adverse outcome, especially deep infection. Although risk of infection for type I injuries approach the same rates as closed injuries, the rate of infection for type III fractures can range from 10% to 50%.[1,2]

GENERALIZED MANAGEMENT PRINCIPLES

Patients generally sustain open fractures of the foot and ankle region from high-energy trauma. Concomitant injuries can be present and should be sought. A thorough evaluation should be performed using advanced trauma life support (ATLS) principles.

The presence of an open wound adjacent to a bony injury signifies an open, or compound, fracture. Plain radiographs of the injured area as well as the joint above and below should be obtained in the anteroposterior and lateral projection. Unfortunately, patients with open injuries are often in significant pain, positioning of the limb is difficult, and can result in less than optimal imaging, compromising establishing an accurate diagnosis and instituting a proper treatment regimen.

General principles of open fracture management have evolved over time. Many recommendations have developed based on military experience. Current clinical guidelines mirror those established by policies enforced in the Korean and Vietnam conflicts. These guidelines include the following:

1. Immobilize the injured extremity and apply sterile dressing to the wound
2. Administer early intravenous antibiotics

3. Perform urgent operative wound debridement and irrigation
4. Stabilize skeletal injury
5. Perform repeat debridement as necessary
6. Delay wound closure/coverage

These principles provide a framework to help the clinician manage an open fracture. Certainly, each injury must be assessed on a case-by-case basis. There has been recent literature demonstrating satisfactory results with early, but by no means urgent, debridement.[3] Immediate wound closure in clean, low-energy wounds, especially type I, II, and some IIIa, has gained clinical acceptance.[4] Clean, low-energy wounds likely highlight the difference between combat and civilian wounds.

Initial treatment in the emergency department plays a key role in the successful management of open fractures about the foot and ankle. At the author's institution, after the diagnosis is established with radiographs and clinical examination, the wound is irrigated with a saline solution to remove gross contamination, and the limb is realigned with a combination of traction and manipulation. A sterile dressing and well-padded sugar-tong and/or posterior splint are applied. A thorough neurovascular examination should be performed both prereduction and postreduction. Additional radiographs of the protected limb can now be obtained. For complex injuries, additional studies can be considered, such as computed tomographic (CT) scans. CT scans provide improved imaging of the bony damage and are particularly useful in intra-articular fractures and injuries to the hind-foot and mid-foot.

Antibiotic delivery should be started as soon as the diagnosis is established. Recent evidence suggests that the time to antibiotic delivery is a key factor in decreasing infection rates, and likely more important than the time to debridement. Antibiotic selection, mode of delivery, and duration are covered elsewhere later in this article.

During the time in the emergency department, patients should be adequately resuscitated and life-threatening and limb-threatening injuries should be identified and addressed. The presence of an open fracture does not necessarily decompress the limb, and compartment syndrome can be present. Signs and symptoms of compartment syndrome should be sought in any patient with a high-energy injury.

The next 3 sections further elaborate on key issues in the management of open fractures of the foot and ankle, including antibiotic delivery, surgical debridement, and fracture stabilization.

ANTIBIOTIC DELIVERY

Clearly, in 2013, no one would question that antibiotics are necessary in the management of open fractures; this was not always the case. Patzaklo and colleagues[5,6] demonstrated a marked reduction in infection rates with open fractures when cephalothin was administered (2.4%) compared with no antibiotics (13.9%). Since this 1974 prospective, randomized study, many additional authors have confirmed that antibiotics play a significant role in decreasing infection rates with open fractures.

Questions, however, still do remain, including which antibiotic or combination is most appropriate, the mode of delivery (local, systemic, or both), and the duration of use.

Most infections that develop following open fractures are the result of natural skin flora. Therefore, an antibiotic with broad-spectrum gram-positive coverage, such as a first-generation cephalosporin, is given in the emergency department for all type I, II, and III open fractures. Multiagent therapy is generally recommended for type III fractures, with an aminoglycoside added to the cephalosporin. Special considerations are present for barnyard-type injuries with gross contamination or injuries occurring in brackish water. Barnyard injuries are predisposed to infection with *Clostridium perfringens*, which can result in gas gangrene and myonecrosis. Penicillin G should be added to the initial treatment regimen in such injuries. In fractures sustained in brackish water, patients are predisposed to infection with Pseudomonas sp. Additional antibiotic coverage should be provided with a fluoroquinolone or a third-generation or fourth-generation cephalosporin.

Duration of therapy remains unclear. It is recognized that earlier delivery is beneficial in decreasing infection risk. Antibiotics should be started as soon as possible after injury occurs because delay greater than 3 hours has been shown the increase infection rates.[2] Antibiotics are generally continued for 24 to 48 hours after surgical debridement and closure. Antibiotics are restarted with each return to the operating room and continued for an additional 24 to 48 hours after each surgical procedure.[2]

Local delivery of antibiotics at the site of injury also has demonstrated promising results. Antibiotic-impregnated polymethylmethacrylate beads can be inserted into the open fracture wound and sealed with a film barrier. High local concentrations at the fracture milieu can be achieved with vancomycin, tobramycin, and/or gentamycin. Advantages of this technique include (1) high local concentration of antibiotics (20 times greater than intravenous therapy), (2) decreased systemic concentration, and (3) a decreased need for systemic aminoglycosides. This technique is most commonly used for type II or III open fracture wounds in combination with systemic therapy.

SURGICAL DEBRIDEMENT

The timing and urgency of surgical debridement have been brought into question with recent literature, but in no means questions the importance of a thorough and timely debridement of the fracture site and zone of injury. If the goals of surgical debridement are not well understood and appreciated, a suboptimal procedure will follow; this places the patient at risk for development of deep infection and ultimately hardware failure.

Goals of debridement include the following:

1. Extend the traumatic wound to visualize the entirety of the zone of injury
2. Explore the wound; identify and remove foreign material
3. Evaluate the local tissue; remove necrotic and nonviable tissue
4. Diminish bacterial contamination
5. Create a stable wound

The traumatic wound is generally extended to visualize the zone of injury, including the skin, subcutaneous fat, muscle, and contaminated bone ends. Wound extension generally continues in a proximal-distal direction until healthy viable tissues are encountered and there is no further periosteal stripping. When extending the open fracture wounds, surgeons often must be creative, but cognizant of the need for future surgical exposure for definitive reconstruction. Devitalized skin and jagged wounds can be ellipsed, but this must be done with great caution in areas where skin is at a premium, such as the foot and ankle.

The entire wound should be carefully inspected. It is often best to take a stepwise approach to the debridement to ensure a meticulous, thorough cleaning has been accomplished. There is likely not a gold standard for how to perform a debridement. However, each surgeon should develop their own routine that can be carefully followed each and every time to ensure a thorough debridement occurs. The simplest method may be to work from outside to the inside. The procedure begins with an inspection of the skin and dermis, followed by subcutaneous fat, muscle, and then bone.

As mentioned previously, necrotic skin edges can be debrided sharply. Local tissues can sometimes be mobilized to overcome the loss of skin and dermis and obtain a primary closure. Unfortunately, injuries resulting in significant skin loss or overly aggressive debridement may result in a wound that requires some type of coverage; this is especially true about the foot and ankle. As a general guideline, skin that is clearly nonviable should be removed, but any skin that is marginal should be left, particularly around the foot and ankle. There is little to no harm in preserving marginal skin with plans for a second-look procedure in 48 to 72 hours.

Debridement of muscle and fascia should generally be more aggressive than the skin. Muscle debridement, in particular, is governed by the mantra, "when in doubt, take it out." Necrotic or damaged muscle serves as the main breeding ground for invading bacteria.

The final step of the debridement consists of delivering the fractured bone edges into the wound. Each end of the bone should be carefully inspected and debrided, including the intramedullary canal. A curette can be used to explore the canal and remove debris. Contaminated bone edges can be removed with a rongeur. Determination of bone viability is often difficult. Unless grossly contaminated, initial bone debridement can be conservative.

IRRIGATION

After adequate debridement has been accomplished, the wound is irrigated, aiming to remove any remaining loose, nonviable tissue and decrease bacterial contamination. Irrigation procedures are governed by the mantra, "dilution is the solution to pollution."

Questions remain regarding the best practice guidelines in regard to volume of irrigation, type of fluid, and mode of delivery. As with the method of debridement, it is likely more important to establish a standardized routine and follow it on each and every case without cutting corners.

How much irrigation? "Dilution is the solution to pollution." "If a little is good, more must be better." Gustilo and Anderson[1] recommended that 10 L of normal saline be used to help diminish risk of infection associated with open fractures. The goals of the irrigation component of the procedure are to remove loose, necrotic tissue and diminish bacterial contamination. Clearly, it goes to reason that the more one irrigates, the more these goals will be met. Authorities generally recommend at least 9 L of irrigant for type III fractures.[7]

Normal saline remains the standard irrigant at most institutions. Several antiseptics have been studied as additives to the saline solution, including hydrogen peroxide, chlorhexidine, and iodine. It was postulated that these agents would further diminish bacterial loads, as they have been shown to be bacteriocidal. They inhibit bacteria by damaging the cell walls. Unfortunately, these agents are also toxic to the host and have been shown to lead to impaired osteoblast function, delayed wound healing, and cartilage damage. Use of these agents is not supported by current literature. The addition of antibiotic to the saline irrigant also has not demonstrated clear clinical benefit.[7]

Multiple modes of delivery are available, including pulsatile lavage, gravity-flow irrigation, bulb syringe, and Waterpik systems. Pulsatile lavage has multiple benefits. It results in improved mobilization of particulate matter and removes such debris from the wound bed. A high volume of fluid can be delivered over a shorter time frame. It results in dramatic decreases in surface bacterial load. Anglen and colleagues[8] demonstrated a 100-fold decrease in bacterial count of Staphylococcus with pulsatile lavage as compared with bulb irrigation. Bhandari and colleagues[9] demonstrated that pulsatile lavage could remove up to 99% of surface bacteria. Recent concerns have arisen regarding the deleterious effects of the pulsatile lavage. Authors have proposed that the high-pressure flow may result in damage to the bone and surrounding soft tissue, resulting in delayed fracture healing. It is also thought that the high-pressure flow may actually force contaminants and bacteria deeper within the tissues, clearly an undesirable outcome. Concerns regarding the use of pulse lavage have led to support for other modes of delivery, such as the Waterpik, surface irrigant systems, or gravity-flow irrigation systems.

At the author's institution, irrigation is generally carried out with 9 L of normal saline using a pulsatile lavage system for type III fractures. In most cases, a thorough debridement is first performed, followed by 6 L of irrigation. At this point, a second-look debridement is performed, followed by a final 3 L of irrigation. For type I and II fractures, 6 L of irrigation is used, with a second-look debridement performed after irrigation with the first 3 L bag of normal saline. Certainly, there are exceptions to every rule. Highly contaminated open fractures may require additional irrigation at the discretion of the surgeon.

TIMING OF DEBRIDEMENT

Emergent debridement of open fractures within a 6-hour window has long been thought necessary to prevent development of infection. The origin of this gold standard likely dates back to 1898, when Paul Leopold Friedrich[10] demonstrated the importance of surgical debridement in a guinea pig model contaminated with garden mold and dust from stairs. Friedrich demonstrated that the initial phases of bacterial growth lasted about 6 to 8 hours after inoculation; this represented the time frame in which surgical debridement appeared the most successful. Clearly, modern medicine has come a long way since the time of Friedrich and 1898. In 2014, there are more aggressive methods of surgical debridement and irrigation, improved resuscitation of the injured patient, and timely delivery of potent systemic antibiotics.

In 1976, Gustilo and Anderson[1] concluded that there is universal agreement that open fractures require urgent debridement and irrigation of the wound. Their stance was not supported by any comparative data, but rather presented as an opinion.

Since that time, many studies have examined the time frame from injury to surgical debridement and the effect of delay on outcomes and risk of infection. Most have been unable to demonstrate an increased risk of infection with delays in debridement from 6 to 24 hours postinjury. There are no level I studies comparing early and delayed surgical debridement for open fractures.

Bednar and Parikh[11] analyzed 75 patients with 82 open fractures. Time from injury to debridement averaged 8.8 hours. There was delay greater than 6 hours in 62 of 82 fractures. Patients were grouped into 6-hour blocks for the first 24 hours. There was no apparent advantage in regard to decreased infection rate in those patients taken to the operating room within 6 hours.

In 2003, Kathod and colleagues[12] analyzed 106 open fractures in 103 patients. Infection rate correlated strongly with increasing Gustilo fracture type. No difference was shown in infection rates based on time from injury to initial surgical debridement.

Spencer and colleagues[13] conducted a prospective study to determine if delay of greater than 6 hours to debridement would lead to increased infection rates. Sixty percent of patients underwent debridement within 6 hours. The other 40% comprised a second group. Infection rates were 10.1% and 10.8%, respectively.

Noumi and colleagues[14] retrospectively analyzed 89 open fractures in 88 patients. Time to debridement was divided into 2 groups (<6 hours or >6 hours). Time from injury to debridement was not determined to be an independent risk factor for infection; Gustilo fracture type was.

The LEAP study[15] reviewed timing of treatment in 315 patients with open fractures. These patients all sustained limb-threatening lower extremity fractures. No significant relationship was established between time to debridement and development of infection. However, time from injury to admission to definitive treatment center was shown to correlate with infection risk. Proposed mechanisms to support this link include aggressive patient resuscitation and delivery of systemic antibiotics.

Other authors have published data supporting the 6-hour rule and the need for urgent surgical debridement.

In reality, the delay from injury to surgery is often multifactorial. Open fractures can occur in isolation or may be part of a constellation of injuries. They may be considered the main priority for the patient or of little immediate importance in patients with life-threatening injuries. Patients may require initial resuscitation and management of more serious injuries before contemplating a trip to the operating room for irrigation and debridement of an open fracture. Patients may present to a smaller institution without the resources to manage complex open fractures. In these cases, it may be beneficial to start antibiotics at the transferring facility, based on the results of the LEAP study. Delays in time from injury to surgical debridement may be due to transfer from a smaller institution to one readily equipped to deal with severe musculoskeletal injury. Operating room availability may present another challenge, especially in those patients arriving to the emergency department at certain hours.

In conclusion, there is little support in the literature to mandate an urgency to surgical debridement following an open fracture. Improved resuscitation and early delivery of systemic antibiotics allow for open fractures to be managed with a timely thorough debridement. Patients should be thoroughly evaluated and concomitant injuries should be excluded or treated appropriately before proceeding to the operating room. Unless this is carried out, proceeding with emergent debridement may pose unjustified risks to the patient.

At the author's institution, open fractures are generally taken to the operating room in a timely manner. Most irrigation and debridement procedures can be safely delayed to daytime hours when there is operating room and surgeon availability. It is thought to be beneficial to the patient and the system as a whole. A fracture specialist who will provide the definitive care for the fracture, rather than an on-call provider, generally carries out the procedure, thus eliminating concerns with inadequate debridement, poor incision placement, and inappropriately placed temporary hardware. It also unburdens the nighttime operating room staff to care for more emergent conditions. Prolonged unnecessary delays to the debridement procedure certainly are not advocated; most patients undergo surgery within 12 hours and all within 24 hours unless there are life-threatening injuries preventing the patient from going to the operating room. These patients are generally managed with a bedside lavage and splinting or traction. Each institution has different capabilities and resources. The key in managing these injuries is establishing protocols and following them accordingly.

SKELETAL STABILIZATION

In most cases, open fractures require some form of skeletal stabilization. Recommendations for specific injuries are provided in later sections. However, there are common goals for all fracture patterns.

1. It is important to restore length and alignment to the limb. This restoration has multiple benefits, including improving vascular and lymphatic flow. The fracture pattern

is often better understood, especially in complex open tibial plafond fractures. Restoring normal anatomy will help eliminate dead space, which can be a source of hematoma and bacterial proliferation. By restoring length and alignment, the extent of the wound and potential need for soft tissue coverage are often better appreciated. There are centers that will maintain certain injuries in a deformed position to obtain primary closure and later regain length and alignment with Ilizarov techniques; this is the exception, rather than the rule.

2. As in all fractures, it is important to strive for anatomic articular reduction. Anatomic articular reduction can generally be accomplished early if the articular surface is easily accessed through the open fracture wound. If the articular injury is simple and the wound is clean, immediate fixation with lag screws should be considered.

3. Early fixation improves wound access. Application of large bulky splints and dressings makes wound inspection and access difficult. Fracture stabilization with either internal or external fixation devices will allow ease of wound care.

4. Fracture stability improves overall patient care. It becomes difficult to move patients with unstable limbs to different areas of the hospital for necessary care and testing.

In reality, there is no gold standard in regard to methods of skeletal stabilization in open fracture management. Each injury represents a unique scenario, with varying degrees of skin, soft tissue, and bony injury. It is important to be familiar with multiple techniques of fracture stabilization, ranging from simple (ie, splinting, pins) to complex (internal/external fixation).

Splinting and casting remain safe, simple, and effective techniques. Commonly, splints are applied in the emergency department and used as a temporary means of stabilization before taking the patient to the operating room. For type I and simple type II open wounds associated with nondisplaced fractures, splints and casts can be considered as a means of definitive care.

External fixation techniques offer many advantages in the management of open fractures, as follows: (1) they can provide adequate, often excellent, stability and realign the major fracture fragments; (2) they are easily and rapidly applied; (3) minimal incisions are required, which are distant from the zone of injury. Therefore, no further soft tissue dissection or periosteal stripping is required at the fracture site; (4) these devices can be used as definitive or temporary fixation. Use of external fixation as a temporary fixation device has gained popularity in the management of complex high-energy fractures of the lower extremities. They allow mobilization of the patient and improved care of the open wounds. Additional testing, including CT scans, can be obtained in the frame to allow for improved preoperative planning. When using the external fixator as a means of temporary fixation, there are several principles to follow. These principles are extremely important, because the surgeon applying the external fixator is often not the one providing the definitive reconstruction. Lack of adherence to basic principles may compromise ultimate fixation and patient outcome. Before application of the fixator, thorough irrigation and debridement are imperative. When planning placement of the fixator, gentle traction should be applied to the limb, and the extent of fracture in a proximal-distal direction should be visualized on fluoroscopy and marked on the skin. An initial plan for definitive reconstruction should be formulated and skin incisions or extensions of the open fracture wound needed for reconstruction should be marked on the skin. There is theoretic concern that pins placed in areas of future incisions or hardware placement will lead to increased infection rates. Increased infection rates have not been definitively shown, but it is likely the best practice to place pins far enough away from injury site to avoid planned hardware placement and incisions. After placement of pins and bars, clamps should be loosely tightened after applying traction. Reduction should be checked with biplanar fluoroscopy. At this time, reduction can be fine-tuned under fluoroscopic guidance while loosening and tightening the connection clamps. The best possible reduction should be obtained, because this will make definitive reconstruction easier.

Historically, use of internal fixation in the management of open fractures has been done with great caution because of concerns of infection. However, support for immediate or delayed internal fixation has been growing in the past 30 years with improved overall care, including antibiotics, wound management, and advances in fixation techniques. Each fracture and wound has its own personality and the surgeon must use their own judgment in making a decision regarding fixation techniques. In general, it is likely safe to proceed with immediate internal fixation for simple fracture patterns in clean wound environments. In general, most type I and II open fractures can be managed with immediate open reduction and internal fixation (ORIF), as long as the wound is thought to be clean and immediate or early closure can be obtained. Literature supports immediate ORIF of type III articular fractures of the ankle.[16,17] Temporary external fixation with delayed ORIF or definitive external fixation should be considered in complex fracture patterns and in wounds with significant contamination.

WOUND MANAGEMENT

Similar to management of the bony injury, wound management in open fractures has become more aggressive. Traditionally, wartime management protocols stressed the importance of open wound management with delayed closure or coverage. These protocols have been challenged and may no longer apply to most open civilian fractures. Most type I and II fractures can be managed with immediate closure without concern of dramatic increase in infection rates. Most type III fractures and those with significant contamination are best managed with open techniques and delayed closure or coverage.

One of the primary objectives of managing open fractures is preventing infection. Most acute infections appear to be due to hospital-acquired pathogens. The prominent role of hospital-acquired bacteria in wound infection supports early wound closure/coverage. Considering the multiple aggressive pathogens present in a hospital setting, the open fracture wound may be cleanest after the initial irrigation and debridement.

One of the early objectives in managing open fractures is obtaining coverage of the bone and soft tissues with skin or some viable alternative. Primary closure seems advantageous because it converts an open wound into a closed one. However, wounds must meet certain criteria to be considered for immediate primary closure:

1. The original wound was relatively clean
2. The place of injury was not grossly contaminated (ie, barnyard)
3. Debridement successfully removed all necrotic tissue and debris
4. The patient's overall condition is satisfactory
5. The wound can be closed without tension

If these criteria are not met, it is likely best to use open management techniques. Very little literature is available regarding the timing of closure for open fracture wounds.

Benson and colleagues[18] compared primary closure (44 wounds) versus delayed closure at an average of 6 days (38 wounds) in regard to infection rates. Superficial infection developed in 3 immediate closure patients. Deep infection developed in 2 patients with delayed closure. No difference was present statistically.

Delong and colleagues[19,20] reviewed 119 open fractures wounds managed with multiple coverage techniques, including immediate closure. Statistical analysis demonstrated no difference in infection rates between immediate and delayed closure groups.

Despite support for immediate closure, concern remains regarding development of anaerobic infection and gas gangrene. Brown and Kinman[20] documented multiple cases of clostridial wound infection in wounds closed primarily. These clostridial wound infections were all severely contaminated wounds, with foreign material including dirt and vegetative matter remaining in the wounds at time of debridement for infection. The authors cautioned against early closure. In reality, this article more likely highlights the need for aggressive thorough debridement and the importance of careful selection of wounds amenable to primary closure.

In conclusion, surgical judgment is necessary to use an immediate closure protocol for open fracture wounds. Most type I and II and some type IIIa wounds may be amenable to immediate closure. Obvious exceptions remain including wounds grossly contaminated with dirt, feces, or stagnant water. If doubt exists, leave the wound open and return to the operating room in 48 to 72 hours for a second look. In areas where skin and soft tissue are at a premium, such as the foot and ankle, leaving a wound completely open may allow the skin to retract/contract and doom the patient to a coverage procedure. It is not unreasonable to approximate the skin edges and return to the operating in 24 to 48 hours.

For wounds not amenable to immediate closure because of contamination or the degree of skin and soft tissue loss, several options exist.

Delayed primary closure refers to the technique of primary closure obtained by day 5. Basic science has demonstrated that wound healing mechanisms proceed for the first 5 days regardless of whether the wound is closed or not. Therefore, a wound closed by the fifth day will be similar in strength at day 14 to one closed immediately. Management of the wound in the interim can include wet-dry dressing, packing, bead pouch techniques, and negative pressure wound therapy. This strategy allows for repeat irrigation and debridement of the wound and minimizes the risk of anaerobic infection.

When immediate closure or delayed primary closure is not possible because of skin and soft tissue loss, the wound must be covered by alternative strategies.

In wounds with a vascularized soft tissue bed, split-thickness skin grafts provide the best option for coverage. Results are best when grafts are placed on a healthy muscle bed or well-formed granulation tissue. Split-thickness skin grafts do not take well when placed on bare tendons or bone not covered by periosteum.

If there is profound soft tissue defect and exposed bone, flap coverage becomes necessary. Flap coverage is generally not done at the time of initial debridement, but can be. In essence, a free tissue transfer turns an open fracture into a well-vascularized closed one. The work of Godina[21] demonstrated that free tissue transfer within the first 72 hours after injury provided superior results, with earlier bone healing and decreased rates of infection. Gopal and colleagues[22] reported their results with a "fix-and-flap" technique for open tibia fractures. Their goal was to obtain coverage within 72 hours. Sixty-three fractures were categorized as the early coverage group; 21 patients were categorized as delayed. Deep infection rates were 6% for early flap and 30% for those with late flaps.

OPEN ANKLE FRACTURES

Fractures of the distal tibia and fibula represent a wide spectrum of injuries. Rotational injuries often lead to spiral distal-third tibial shaft and fibular shaft fractures or malleolar fractures. Forceful axial loads often result in severe comminuted fractures of the tibial plafond and distal fibula with severe soft tissue damage.

Rotational ankle fractures generally result from lower energy injuries (**Fig. 1**). Typical fracture patterns include bimalleolar fractures, trimalleolar fractures, or bimalleolar equivalent fractures, with deltoid ligament incompetence. The ankle joint itself is usually dislocated with open injuries and the syndesmosis is often injured. The typical wound pattern is a transverse medial wound. These wounds are often amenable to immediate closure, although caution should be used in grossly contaminated wounds.

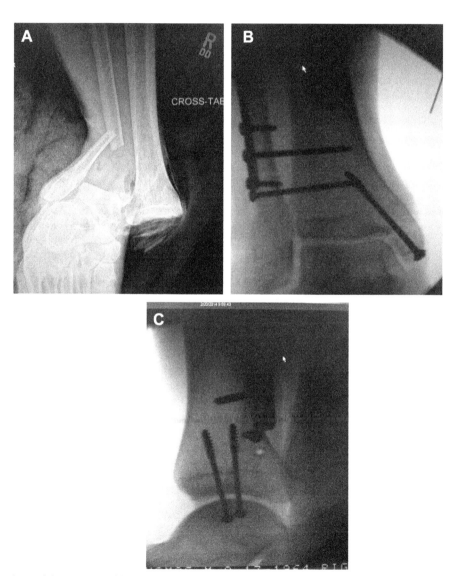

Fig. 1. (*A*) A 39-year-old man with grade 3 bimalleolar fracture and syndesmostic injury. (*B*) Immediate debridement and ORIF of bimalleolar fracture and syndesmotic disruption. (*C*) Lateral radiograph following immediate ORIF.

The fracture pattern dictates operative needs. In general, these fractures can undergo immediate reduction and fixation. Delayed definitive care can be considered in grossly contaminated wounds or if the operative surgeon is not comfortable with standard fixation techniques. In these cases, debridement followed by splinting or placement of an ankle spanning external fixator can be considered.

After thorough irrigation and debridement, the wound should be assessed. If clean, immediate reduction and fixation are carried out. The open fracture wound is often medial. The medial injury can be addressed through the open fracture wound and typically consists of a transverse medial malleolar fracture or complete rupture of deltoid ligament. Medial malleolar fractures should be reduced anatomically and stabilized with 2 lag screws. Generally, 3.5-mm cortical or 4.0-mm partially threaded screws are used. Cannulated screws can be considered, but are often not necessary because of the added cost. If the injury is a deltoid ligament rupture, lateral fixation must be carried out first. At this point, it is often beneficial to repair the medial soft tissues back to bone with suture anchors or through drill holes. In closed fractures, the deltoid ligament injury is typically ignored and allowed to heal at its normal resting length. However, in open wounds, it seems logical that this component of the injury complex should be addressed as well, because it can be accomplished without further extension of the open wound. The fibula fracture is addressed though a separate, longitudinal lateral incision. Standard techniques of fixation are used. In general, oblique fractures are first reduced and stabilized by 2.7-mm or 3.5-mm lag screws. After lag screw placement, a lateral one-third tubular neutralization plate is applied with at least 2 points of fixation on each side of the fracture. At this point, any syndesmotic injury or posterior malleolar fracture can be addressed. Posterior malleolar fractures can generally be visualized on the preoperative imaging studies. Any fracture comprising greater than 20% of the articular surface generally requires fixation. In open fractures, the posterior component can usually be clamped through the medial open wound and stabilized with anterior-posterior lag screws. Other methods of fixation include posterior to anterior screws or a posterior applied plate. After fractures are stabilized, the stability of the syndesmosis should be assessed. Syndesmotic instability is often easy to visualize on preoperative imaging with the ankle dislocated. However, more subtle instability should not be ignored. It is recommended that a stress examination (ie, cotton test) be performed on all ankle fractures under live fluoroscopic imaging. Syndesmotic reduction and fixation are carried out through the lateral wound. Obtaining an anatomic reduction is often difficult, as authors have documented a high prevalence of malreduction of syndesmotic injuries. Stabilization techniques are also controversial. In general, screw placement is generally carried out in a slightly posterior to anterior direction with the ankle in a neutral position. Controversy exists as to whether 1 or 2 screws are adequate, whether 3 or 4 cortices of fixation are better, and if screws should be 3.5 mm or 4.5 mm in diameter. Following fixation, stability of the ankle joint itself should be assessed. For bimalleolar or trimalleolar fractures, surgical repair of the fractures and suture repair of the ankle capsule and wound itself with the joint reduced often provide adequate stability to manage the limb in a well-padded splint. For patients with significant instability, particularly those with a medial ligamentous disruption, consideration should be given to placement of a medial ankle spanning external fixator.

Open fractures of the tibial plafond result from high-energy injuries and are usually associated with significant comminution of the distal tibia and soft tissue injury (**Figs. 2 and 3**). Location of the open wound is typically medial, but can be variable. Treatment should proceed with debridement of the wound and thorough assessment of the

473

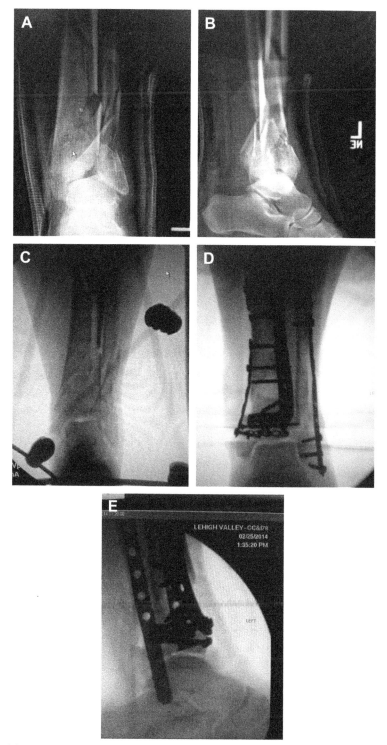

Fig. 2. (*A*) Comminuted grade II open tibial plafond fracture. (*B*) Preoperative lateral radiograph. (*C*) Placement of ankle spanning external fixator for staged management of open pilon fracture. (*D*) Postoperative anteroposterior (AP) radiograph demonstrating satisfactory reduction. (*E*) Postoperative lateral radiograph demonstrating satisfactory reduction.

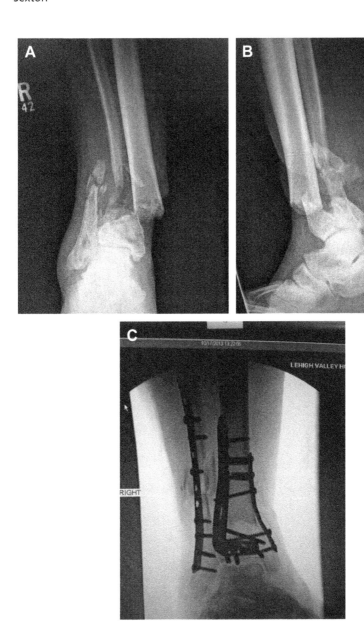

Fig. 3. (A) Comminuted grade 2 open pilon fracture. (B) Injury lateral radiograph of tibial plafond fracture. (C) Delayed reconstruction of comminuted pilon fracture.

fracture pattern. In a clean wound that appears amenable to immediate closure with a simple fracture pattern, immediate fixation can be considered with acceptable complication rates. Fixation should proceed through extension of the open fracture wound with direct anatomic reduction of the articular component of the fracture with indirect reduction of the metaphyseal component of the injury. For complex fractures or wounds not amenable to immediate closure or with gross contamination, staged fixation strategies should be used. A joint spanning fixator is applied with or without immediate fixation of the fibula through a posterolateral incision. If the fibula fracture pattern is simple and the fixation is to be performed by the surgeon planning on doing the definitive reconstruction, immediate fixation through a posterolateral incision will be beneficial in restoring length and alignment to the limb. If the fibula fracture is comminuted and reduction will be difficult, it may be best to delay fibular fixation until the time of the definitive procedure. Malreduction of the fibular will make reduction of the tibial plafond difficult, if not impossible. Satisfactory outcomes can be expected in most type I and II open fractures. For type III open plafond fractures, there remains a high rate of complications, including deep infection and nonunion. For fractures with severe soft tissue loss requiring free flap coverage, it is generally best to perform internal fixation at the same time as flap coverage.

The use of external fixation has a role in both the acute and the definitive management of tibial plafond fractures. Authors have shown satisfactory results with the use of external fixation as definitive management with or without limited internal fixation of the articular surface.

OPEN HIND-FOOT INJURIES

There is a paucity of skin and soft tissue overlying the hind-foot. Open injuries often result in exposed bone, tendon, or cartilage. Timely coverage is necessary to promote an environment conducive to healing. Many open wounds in this region can be managed successfully with primary or delayed primary closure. Extensive tissue loss may require free tissue transfer, because there are limited local flaps available with the possible exception of a sural-based flap. The ultimate goal is to obtain soft tissue coverage/closure in a timely manner, with durable, functional, and esthetic coverage.

Heel pad avulsion injuries represent a special type of injury. Although there is not a fracture, this injury pattern requires aggressive management and often leads to poor outcomes. The heel pad is a unique structure with biomechanical properties that cannot be replicated. This tissue is capable of withstanding significant shear and compression forces during standing and walking. These injuries are best addressed with timely irrigation and debridement with attempts at primary repair. Flap survival depends on retrograde blood flow and often cannot be predicted at the time of the initial procedure. The author generally attempts to reattach the fibroelastic tissue back to the calcaneus, from which it is avulsed. This reattachment of the fibroelastic tissue can be accomplished with sutures placed through the bone or suture anchors. Skin closure should then be accomplished without tension.

Open injuries to the hind-foot result from a variety of mechanisms. Calcaneal fractures generally follow a significant axial load, resulting in a comminuted, intra-articular fracture. The soft tissue defect may occur from a bone spike penetration from inside out or tearing of the subcutaneous tissues due to fracture deformity. In calcaneal fractures, the primary fracture line results in separation of the middle facet from the tuberosity and in shortening and lateral translation of the tuberosity fragment in relationship to the sustentaculum, creating tension on the medial skin and subcutaneous tissue, which can lead to tearing and an open wound. Alternatively, the sharp spike of the sustentaculum may penetrate the medial skin. Based on these factors, the open wound is usually at the medial hind-foot. Pathomechanics of talar neck and body fractures and peritalar dislocations are harder to characterize. Neck fractures generally occur when a load is applied with the ankle dorsiflexed. There is generally a medial-sided compression and lateral sided tension failure. Wound location is variable.

Goals of treatment of open hind-foot injuries are similar to other open fractures. These treatments include timely irrigation and debridement of the open wound, early antibiotic delivery, restoration of normal alignment of the bony architecture with internal or external fixation, timely coverage or wound closure, and minimizing the rate of complications. Unfortunately, some of these injuries are so severe and soft tissue loss so great that timely recognition of an unsalvageable limb is also important. A timely amputation may be more beneficial to the patient than an attempt at salvage and multiple surgical procedures.

The decision for timing of definitive fixation of these injuries is debatable. Many factors, including the size, location, and degree of contamination of the wound, fracture pattern and severity, surgeon experience, and medical status of the patient, play a role. Calcaneal fractures, with a typical medial-based wound, will undergo a timely debridement procedure with reduction of the fracture. Definitive fixation can be delayed until resolution of soft tissue swelling with plans for an extensile lateral approach or proceed early if fixation can be obtained through the open medial wound for certain fracture patterns. Open talar fracture-dislocation is often reduced and stabilized immediately.

Talar neck and body fractures typically result from high-energy injuries in younger patients (see **Fig. 3**). Open injuries suggest even more significant soft tissue and bony injury than their closed counterparts. Talar neck fractures can be differentiated from body fractures based on the location of the fracture line. Neck fractures are extra-articular and the fracture line does not violate the posterior facet of the subtalar joint. Conversely, body fractures extend into the ankle joint, subtalar joint, or both.

Open talar neck fractures require timely irrigation and debridement. These fractures can be stabilized at the initial procedure granted that there exists a clean wound bed and the surgeon is comfortable in managing talus fractures. If not, there are no studies proving that ultimate outcome is less satisfactory with staged fixation, providing the fracture is provisionally reduced and temporary stabilization is obtained. Temporary stability can be obtained with K-wires or spanning external fixation. If immediate fixation is selected, fracture reduction can be accomplished through extension of the open fracture wound. Often, a second incision is required for confirmation of reduction and application of additional fixation (**Fig. 4**). Talar neck fractures often have medial comminution, suggesting a varus moment during injury. The medial comminution makes anatomic reduction difficult to obtain through the medial wound. A second anterolateral approach allows for visualization of lateral aspect of the talar neck fracture, where tensile failure has occurred, allowing for confirmation of anatomic reduction and prevention of varus malunion. Utilization of the second incision must be done with caution, based on the degree of soft tissue injury and surgeon experience. Fracture fixation can be accomplished via the use of lag screw technique or plate-and-screw constructs. For fractures with significant medial comminution, plate-and-screw constructs may be preferable as compression obtained with lag screw fixation may promote varus malunion (**Fig. 5**).

Open talar body fractures can be stabilized during the initial debridement procedure. However, these injuries are often managed in a delayed fashion. Temporary fixation can often be obtained with reduction of the fragments and placement in a splint. If significant soft tissue injury exists or the ankle remains unstable, a temporary spanning external fixator can be applied. Once soft tissue swelling improves and fracture blisters heal, a definitive reconstruction can be planned and performed based on plain imaging and CT scans. A medial malleolar and/or lateral malleolar osteotomy are often required to obtain anatomic reduction and place fixation in comminuted talar body fractures (**Fig. 6**).

Talar neck and body fractures represent significant injuries. Good and excellent outcomes are hard to obtain in closed injuries and unlikely in open injuries. The goals in treating these high-energy injuries are to provide the patient with a functional lower

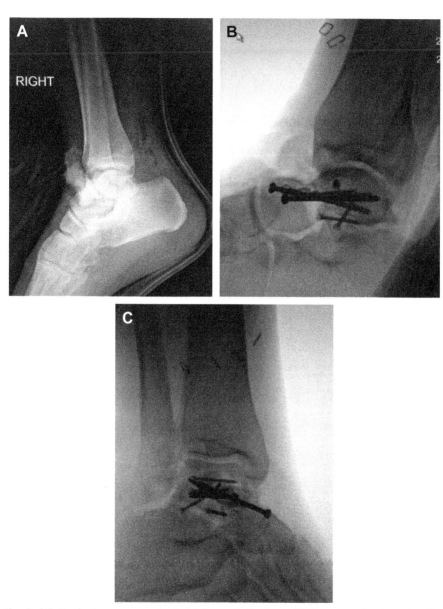

Fig. 4. (*A*) Grade 2 open comminuted talar neck fracture. (*B*) Postoperative lateral radiograph demonstrating satisfactory reduction after staged fixation of talar neck fracture. (*C*) AP radiograph demonstrating satisfactory reconstruction of complex talus fracture.

extremity, obtain union of the fractures, and avoid infection. Osteonecrosis will occur in up to 50% of displaced talar neck fractures.[23] The rate is lower for talar body fractures, but there is a high incidence of posttraumatic ankle and subtalar arthritis. Deep infection is unfortunately quite common after these open injuries and leads to poor outcome. Marsh and colleagues[24] examined 18 patients with open Hawkins type III and extruded talus injuries and reported an infection rate approaching 40%.

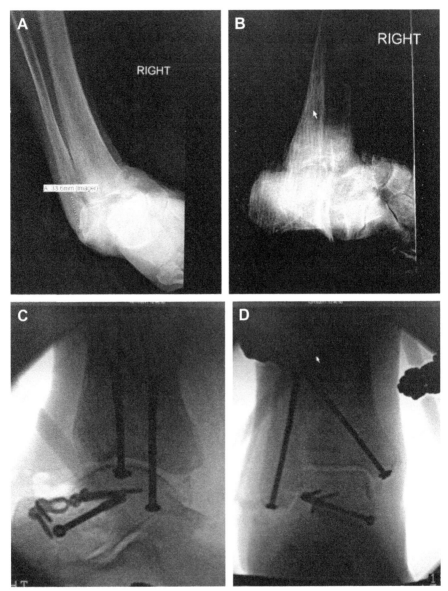

Fig. 5. (A) AP radiograph demonstrating complex talar neck fracture-dislocation. (B) Injury lateral radiograph demonstrating significant displacement. (C) Postoperative lateral radiograph demonstrating immediate fixation of complex injury. (D) Postoperative AP radiograph demonstrating satisfactory reconstruction.

Open peritalar (subtalar) dislocation generally presents with significant deformity and tearing of the joint capsule and overlying tissues. Dislocation can occur in medial or lateral directions. Medial injuries are more common in general, but open injuries tend to be lateral dislocations. There is no general consensus on the best means of treating the bony injury. Basic tenets of open fracture care apply. Obtaining a

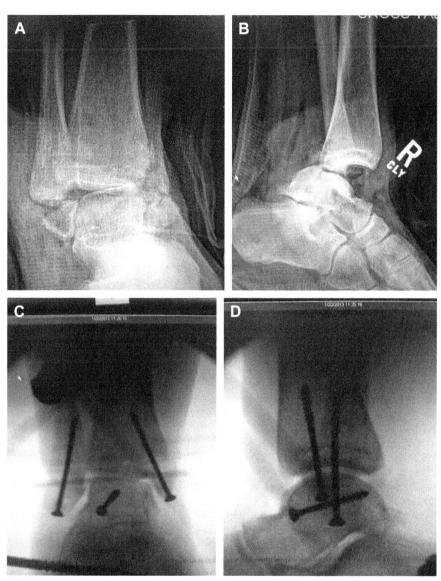

Fig. 6. (*A*) AP radiograph with grade 2 open bimalleolar fracture. (*B*) Lateral radiograph demonstrating additional talar body fracture. (*C*) AP radiograph demonstrating fixation of all fractures. Talar body fracture was fixed first using the malleolar fractures for visualization. Supplemental external fixation was applied. (*D*) Postoperative lateral radiograph demonstrating satisfactory reduction.

reduction is not always easy; multiple impediments exist. Reduction of a lateral dislocation may be blocked by the posterior tibial or flexor digitorum longus tendon or a traumatic talar head defect. The talonavicular joint capsule and the extensor digitorum brevis muscle commonly prevent reduction of a medial dislocation. Once reduction is obtained, stability is assessed. K-wire fixation across the joints or spanning external fixation can be considered. Again, outcomes following these injuries are often unsatisfactory. Goldner and colleagues[25] reported a high incidence of persistent pain and dysfunction in a series of 15 grade III open peritalar dislocations. All patients had either fair or poor outcomes and reported difficulty with stair climbing and walking on uneven ground. Merchan[26] studied 16 patients with open peritalar dislocations; none reported better than a poor result.

The extruded talus represents a rare injury, usually leading to poor outcomes. The extruded talus is often contaminated by significant foreign material. Acute management is controversial. The options include reimplantation versus talectomy. Reimplantation brings with it high rates of infection and osteonecrosis. Talectomy leads to limb-length inequality, deformity, and instability. Because of the rarity of this injury, there is no universal support for any particular technique. All recommendations are based on case reports or series. Assal and Stern[27] reported on 4 cases of reimplantation of an extruded talus without any soft tissue attachment. No significant complications were noted, differing from historical reports, documenting high rates of infection and osteonecrosis. If reimplantation is selected, the talus must be thoroughly cleansed first. It is recommended that it be soaked in an antibiotic solution followed by a mechanical cleansing with pulsatile lavage. Suture repair of surrounding structures and K-wire fixation of the joint may be beneficial. In cases with severe articular injury or gross contamination, talectomy may be preferable and often leads to poor outcomes; early fusion may be considered.

Open calcaneal fractures result from high-energy injuries, with typical fracture comminution and significant fragment displacement. The wound is typically medial, as mentioned previously. Initial irrigation and debridement proceed with extension of the medial fracture wound. Definitive management strategies include immediate fixation through the medial wound or temporary reduction and provisional stabilization with plans for delayed reconstruction through an extensile lateral approach. When using the lateral approach, it is important to delay repair until the soft tissues have recovered from the initial insult. Early[28] recommends surgery at approximately 10 days through a lateral approach if the wound is medial, stable, and less than 4 cm. Benirschke and Kramer[29] noted a 7.7% complication rate with delayed use of the lateral extensile approach in 39 open calcaneal fractures. There is a wide disparity in results documented in the literature. Siebert and colleagues[30] studied 36 open calcaneal fractures retrospectively. Multiple strategies were used for fracture stabilization including nonsurgical. Deep infection occurred in 39% and 5 extremities required amputation (14%). Berry and colleagues[31] also used a variety of techniques to manage 30 open calcaneal fractures. No deep infections were reported. Despite some positive reports, it seems most series suggest a complication rate ranging from 10% to 50%, with negative prognostic factors, including a wound greater than 5 cm in length, presence of neurovascular injury, need for free tissue transfer, presence of heel pad avulsion injury, plantar wound location, and presence of severe comminution.

OPEN MID-FOOT AND LISFRANC INJURIES

Open injuries to the mid-foot, including the navicular, cuboid, and cuneiforms, and Lisfranc disruptions, present a challenge to the treating physician. There is a poor soft tissue envelope and coverage options are limited. These injuries range from type 1 open wounds, which can be managed with standard fixation techniques and immediate closure, to the mangled foot, which may necessitate amputation.

Navicular fractures are generally intra-articular fractures with consistent fracture lines. CT scan imaging may be necessary to understand the fracture patterns. Open treatment with internal fixation and lag screws is typically required for displaced fractures.

Open injuries to the cuneiforms and Lisfranc complex typically present with significant displacement and instability (**Fig. 7**). These injuries can usually be visualized through extension of the open fracture wound. Extent of cartilage damage should be inspected and documented. After debridement, fractures and/or joint dislocations

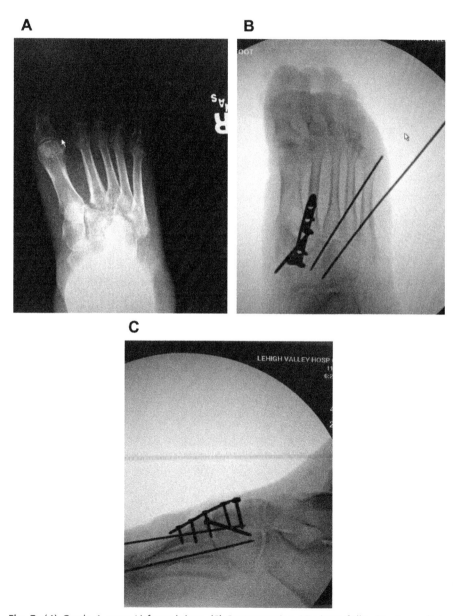

Fig. 7. (*A*) Grade 1 open Lisfranc injury. (*B*) Postoperative AP views following immediate reconstruction and primary closure. (*C*) Postoperative lateral radiograph following fixation of Lisfranc injury.

should be reduced and temporarily stabilized with K-wires or clamps. Depending on the extent of articular damage, there is a role for preparation of the joint surfaces and immediate fusion in these injuries. Definitive fixation can then be accomplished. Typically, in nonfusion cases, positional screws are placed across the injured joint to maintain them in a reduced position. A Lisfranc screw may be placed from the medial cuneiform to the second metatarsal to substitute for the damaged ligament. In fusion cases, lag screw

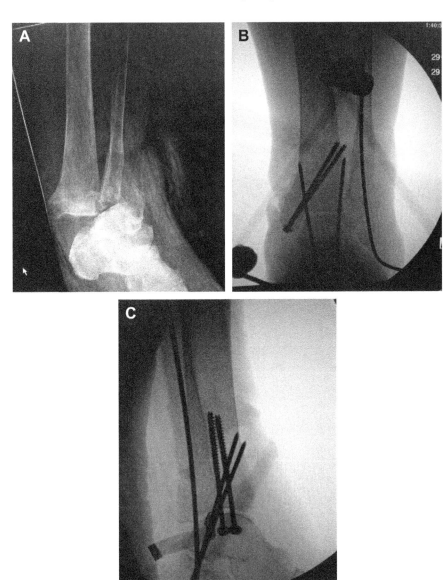

Fig. 8. (A) Complex open ankle fracture dislocation in elderly diabetic patient. (B) AP radiograph demonstrating anatomic reduction with composite fixation including ORIF, pins placed across the tibio-talo-calcaneal joints, and ankle spanning external fixator. (C) Lateral radiograph demonstrating excellent reduction and composite fixation. It is necessary to place pins through the anterior cortex to aid in removal in case they break.

fixation and compression are beneficial. Alternative strategies for stabilization are useful in cases with fractures at the metatarsal bases. Joint bridging mini-fragment plates can be applied over the dorsal joint surfaces from the metatarsal to the cuneiform or navicular if necessary. Timing and need for hardware removal are controversial.

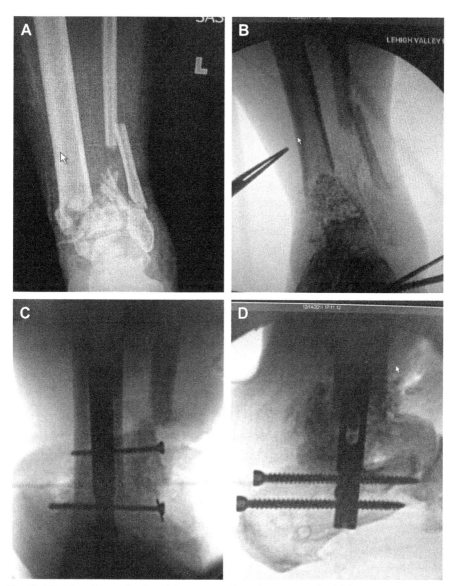

Fig. 9. (*A*) AP radiograph of multitrauma patient that received initial care at an outside facility who presented 1 month after injury with draining wound and loose external fixator. (*B*) Patient underwent debridement, at which time gross purulence, retained foreign material, and necrotic bone were found. External fixator was adjusted, and antibiotic beads were placed. (*C*) Ultimate salvage performed with tibiotalocalcaneal fusion and bone grafting. (*D*) Lateral radiograph demonstrating satisfactory alignment with tibiotalocalcaneal fusion.

Cuboid injuries are uncommon and are usually due to a lateral crush injury. Open injuries are rare in isolation. Treatment goals are to restore normal length to the lateral column of the foot, which can be accomplished with ORIF or external fixation spanning the lateral column of the foot. Custom plates are available that fit the lateral wall of the cuboid.

Crush injuries to the mid-foot result in multiple fractures and severe soft tissue damage. Treatment goals aim at restoring length to the medial and lateral columns of the foot and stabilizing displaced fractures and joint dislocations. Several treatment options exist and depend on the extent of bony and soft tissue injury. Reduction and internal fixation of each injury may be possible, but may require extensive dissection and stripping of soft tissues, compromising chances at obtaining wound closure. Limited techniques can include medial and/or lateral bridge plating or spanning external fixation.

SPECIAL CASES

Open fractures around the foot and ankle in patients with significant comorbidities, such as advanced age, osteoporosis, and diabetes mellitus, present significant challenges. Poor bone quality may lead to failure of fixation and poor outcomes. Composite fixation strategies or a "kitchen sink" approach may be necessary to ensure adequate stability until fracture healing (**Fig. 8**).

SUMMARY

Open fractures of the foot and ankle present a wide spectrum of injuries. Simple fracture patterns with type I or II open wounds often behave like closed injuries and good outcomes can be expected. Complex intra-articular fractures with large contaminated wounds often do poorly with a high rate of complications, including infection and wound-healing issues, nonunion, malunion, osteonecrosis, and posttraumatic arthritis (**Fig. 9**).

Each facility should have their own plan and guidelines in dealing with open fractures of the foot and ankle. If resources are not available, transfer arrangements should be considered. Definitive management should consist of timely delivery of antibiotics and surgical debridement. Fracture stabilization should be individualized to the patient and depends on fracture, wound pattern and surgeon comfort. Wound management is a collaboration between the treating fracture surgeon and the plastic surgeon.

REFERENCES

1. Gustilo RB, Anderson JT. Prevention of infection in the treatment of one thousand and twenty-five open fractures of long bones: retrospective and prospective analysis. J Bone Joint Surg Am 1976;58:453–8.
2. Patzakis MJ, Wilkins J. Factors influencing infection rate in open fracture wounds. Clin Orthop 1989;243:36–40.
3. Pollak A. Timing of debridement of open fractures. J Am Acad Orthop Surg 2006; 14:S48–51.
4. Weitz-Marshall A, Bosse M. Timing of closure of open fractures. J Am Acad Orthop Surg 2002;10:379–84.
5. Patzakis MJ, Harvey JP Jr, Ivler D. The role of antibiotics in the management of open fractures. J Bone Joint Surg Am 1974;56:532–41.

6. Ostermann PA, Seligson D, Henry SL. Local antibiotic therapy for severe open fractures: a review of 1085 consecutive cases. J Bone Joint Surg Br 1995;77:93–7.
7. Anglen JO. Wound irrigation in musculoskeletal injury. J Am Acad Orthop Surg 2001;9:219–26.
8. Anglen J, Apostoles S, Christensen G, et al. The efficacy of various irrigation solutions in removing slime-producing staphylococcus. J Orthop Trauma 1994; 8:390–6.
9. Bhandari M, Schemitsch EH, Adili A, et al. High and low pressure pulsatile lavage of contaminated tibial fractures: an in vitro study of bacterial adherence and bone damage. J Orthop Trauma 1999;13:526–33.
10. Friedrich PL. Die Aseptische Versorgung frischer Wunden. Arch Klin Chir 1898; 57:288–310.
11. Bednar DA, Parikh J. Effect of time delay from injury to primary management on the incidence of deep infection after open fractures of the lower extremities caused by blunt trauma in adults. J Orthop Trauma 1993;7:532–5.
12. Kathod M, Botte MJ, Hoyt DB, et al. Outcomes in open tibia fractures: relationship between delay in treatment and infection. J Trauma 2003;55:949–54.
13. Spencer J, Smith A, Woods D. The effect of time delay on infection in open long-bone fractures: a 5-year prospective audit from a district general hospital. Ann R Coll Surg Engl 2004;86:108–12.
14. Noumi T, Yokoyama K, Ohtsuka H, et al. Intramedullary nailing for open fractures of the femoral shaft: evaluation of contributing factors on deep infection and nonunion using multivariate analysis. Injury 2005;36:1085–93.
15. Pollak AN, Jones AL, et al. Time to definitive treatment significantly influences incidence of infection after open high-energy lower-extremity trauma. Presented at the Annual Scientific Meeting of the Orthopaedic Trauma Association. Salt Lake City (UT), October 9–11, 2003.
16. Bray TJ, Endicott M, Capra SE. Treatment of open ankle fractures: immediate internal fixation versus closed immobilization and delayed fixation. Clin Orthop 1989;240:47–52.
17. Franklin JL, Johnson KD, Hansen ST. Immediate internal fixation of open ankle fractures. J Bone Joint Surg Am 1994;66:1349–56.
18. Benson DR, Riggins RS, Lawrence RM, et al. Treatment of open fractures: a prospective study. J Trauma 1983;23:25–30.
19. Delong WG Jr, Born CT, Wei SY, et al. Aggressive treatment of 119 open fracture wounds. J Trauma 1999;46:1049–54.
20. Brown PW, Kinman PB. Gas gangrene in a metropolitan community. J Bone Joint Surg Am 1974;56:1445–51.
21. Godina M. Early microsurgical reconstruction of complex trauma of the extremities. Plast Reconstr Surg 1986;78:285–92.
22. Gopal S, Majumder S, Batchelor AGB, et al. Fix and flap: the radical orthopaedic and plastic treatment of severe open fractures of the tibia. J Bone Joint Surg Br 2000;82:959–66.
23. Vallier HA, Nork SE, Barei DP, et al. Talar neck fractures: results and outcomes. J Bone Joint Surg Am 2004;86:1616–24.
24. Marsh JL, Saltzman CL, Iverson M, et al. Major open injuries of the talus. J Orthop Trauma 1995;9:371–6.
25. Goldner JL, Poletti SC, Gates HS 3rd, et al. Severe open subtalar dislocations. J Bone Joint Surg Am 1995;77:1075–9.
26. Merchan EC. Subtalar dislocations: long term followup of 39 cases. Injury 1992; 23:97–100.

27. Assal M, Stern R. Total extrusion of the talus. J Bone Joint Surg Am 2004;86: 2726–31.
28. Early JS. Treatment protocol for the management of open intra-articular calcaneal fractures. Tech Foot Ankle Surg 2005;4:31–4.
29. Benirschke SK, Kramer PA. Wound healing complications in closed and open calcaneal fractures. J Orthop Trauma 2004;18:1–6.
30. Siebert CH, Hansen M, Wolter D. Follow-up evaluation of open intra-articular fractures of the calcaneus. Arch Orthop Trauma Surg 1998;117:442–7.
31. Berry GK, Stevens DG, Kreder HJ, et al. Open fractures of the calcaneus: a review of treatment and outcome. J Orthop Trauma 2004;18:202–6.

Diabetic Charcot Neuroarthropathy of the Foot and Ankle with Osteomyelitis

Crystal L. Ramanujam, DPM, MSc[a], John J. Stapleton, DPM[b,c],
Thomas Zgonis, DPM[a,*]

KEYWORDS

- Diabetic neuropathy • Ulceration • Charcot foot • Osteomyelitis • External fixation

KEY POINTS

- Diabetic Charcot neuroarthropathy (CN) of the foot and ankle can lead to major pedal complications, including a severe deformity, ulceration, and potential amputation.
- Concomitant osteomyelitis in the presence of a diabetic CN of the foot and ankle can pose a significant challenge in the diagnosis and treatment of the 2 entities.
- Combined medical and surgical treatment strategies through a multidisciplinary team effort may improve long-term outcomes in this population.

INTRODUCTION

Although osteomyelitis is known as one of the oldest diseases, its presence in the diabetic Charcot neuroarthropathy (CN) of the foot and ankle remains challenging in diagnosis, medical management and surgical reconstruction. The most significant risk factor for diabetic CN and osteomyelitis is the presence of a pre-existing ulceration in a patient with dense peripheral neuropathy,[1] which has been shown to drastically increase the amputation risk.[2] Furthermore, a severely dislocated and unstable diabetic CN of the foot and/or ankle might also be a predisposing factor to development of osteomyelitis. Osteomyelitis among patients with diabetic CN of the foot and ankle is most commonly caused by direct contiguous spread of infection from a local area of ulceration. Hematogenous osteomyelitis, although rare, may also be encountered with both acute and/or chronic diabetic CN.

Acute CN, which clinically manifests as a warm, edematous, and often erythematous foot and/or ankle, can often be mistaken for infection. A high index of suspicion

---

[a] Division of Podiatric Medicine and Surgery, Department of Orthopaedic Surgery, University of Texas Health Science Center at San Antonio, 7703 Floyd Curl Drive MSC 7776, San Antonio, TX 78229, USA; [b] Foot and Ankle Surgery, VSAS Orthopaedics, Lehigh Valley Hospital, 1250 South Cedar Crest Boulevard, Suite # 110, Allentown, PA 18103, USA; [c] Penn State College of Medicine, 500 University Drive, Hershey, PA 17033, USA
* Corresponding author.
E-mail address: zgonis@uthscsa.edu

Clin Podiatr Med Surg 31 (2014) 487–492
http://dx.doi.org/10.1016/j.cpm.2013.12.001   podiatric.theclinics.com
0891-8422/14/$ – see front matter © 2014 Elsevier Inc. All rights reserved.

is needed to accurately diagnose this stage of CN and provide adequate immobilization that can help prevent further periarticular lower extremity subluxations and/or dislocations, which often lead to severe deformities and bony prominences in the later stages of CN. In addition, the overuse of oral or systemic antibiosis for an acute CN event is evident, as it is commonly mistaken for cellulitis. Close patient observation while holding the antibiotic therapy may be required to adequately make the diagnosis of acute CN versus infection. This clinical case scenario creates challenges when the osseous deformity of CN eventually ulcerates and does become infected. Antibiotic administration needs to be considered, particularly when cultures reveal drug-resistant pathogens or when patients have a history of kidney or liver disease.

Patients with chronic diabetic CN of the foot and/or ankle are most commonly encountered in the clinical setting, because these patients often do not notice a deformity until an ulceration develops or deformity impedes their ability to ambulate or wear regular shoe gear. The midfoot, particularly the tarsometatarsal (Lisfranc) joint complex, is the most frequent location for joint collapse and disorganization; however, the hindfoot and ankle are becoming increasingly prevalent locations for CN (**Fig. 1**). Excessive pressure at these areas in the diabetic insensate foot and in the absence of proper off-loading can lead to extensive neuropathic ulcerations and subsequent bone infections. The underlying bone at the ulceration site is exposed to bacteria that invade vascular channels and subsequently increase intraosseous pressure that impedes blood flow and finally leads to ischemic bone necrosis. Impaired immune response, often encountered in diabetic patients along with common comorbidities, has also been implicated in allowing these infections to worsen and further increasing the risk of limb loss.[3] It is also important to mention that osteomyelitis itself can trigger the development of neuropathic osteoarthropathy.[4]

The differentiation between diabetic CN and osteomyelitis often poses a significant problem, because both of these entities present with similar clinical and radiographic findings. Plain radiographs are the first diagnostic imaging tool that health care

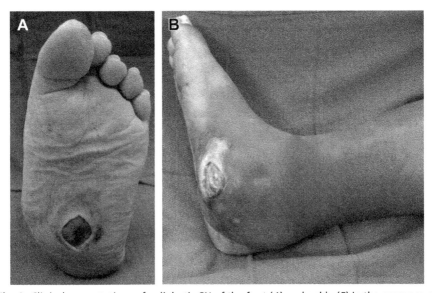

Fig. 1. Clinical presentations of a diabetic CN of the foot (*A*) and ankle (*B*) in the presence of a neuropathic ulceration and concomitant osteomyelitis.

providers should use in evaluating diabetic CN and osteomyelitis. Characteristic changes of osteomyelitis include periosteal reaction, followed by focal cortical or medullary bone erosions; however, these findings can also be found in CN.[5] The introduction of advanced medical imaging has offered additional ways to differentiate osteomyelitis from CN, although with varying degrees of sensitivity and specificity. By the 1970s, nuclear medicine with the use of bone scintigraphy came into widespread use, while the development of technetium-99m-MDP and indium 111-labeled leukocyte tests increased specificity of these imaging techniques for detecting infection. More recently, bone marrow scintigraphy, most commonly sulfur colloid imaging, has become useful in determining CN with and without osteomyelitis.[6] In the 1980s, magnetic resonance imaging (MRI) provided hospitals with another modality to better investigate diabetic foot and ankle infections, and today it is the most used imaging technique for infection. Altered bone marrow signal on MRI is highly sensitive for osteomyelitis, and even in the presence of superimposed CN, these images give excellent anatomic detail and spatial resolution, which is extremely advantageous for operative planning.[5] More recently, since 2000, the positron emission tomography/computed tomography (PET/CT) scan has been used with radiotracers such as fluorodeoxyglucose (FDG), an analogue of glucose, to locate areas of inflammation and infection, providing high spatial resolution. In a study by Keidar and colleagues[7] in 2005, ^{18}F-FDG-labeled white blood cell PET/CT imaging demonstrated promising results for accurate differentiation between diabetic foot osteomyelitis and soft tissue infection. Accurate diagnosis with rapid localization of infection through precise imaging techniques could limit the potential extent of tissue loss and/or amputation during surgical debridement.

Laboratory findings for diabetic CN or osteomyelitis are varied, because most are sensitive but not specific. Leukocytosis may be present, although the often-impaired immune response in diabetic patients can make this an unreliable gauge to measure the severity of infection. Inflammatory markers, erythrocyte sedimentation rate, and C-reactive protein can be useful to monitor response to antibiotic and surgical treatment. Definitive diagnosis for both CN and osteomyelitis is achieved through intraoperative bone biopsy and cultures. Histopathological examination of bone specimens positive for osteomyelitis is most consistent with inflammatory cells, bone marrow changes of fibrosis, reactive bone formation, and trabecular erosions. Positive bacterial growth in bone cultures obtained intraoperatively with susceptibilities is helpful to guide antibiotic therapy.[8] Negative bone cultures cannot rule out osteomyelitis, because this may be caused by the prolonged use of antibiosis given before obtaining the intraoperative bone specimen. Adequate amount and careful handling of all soft tissue and osseous intraoperative specimens should be performed meticulously, because inadequate and contamination of specimens may alter results and complicate further treatment planning.

For diabetic CN of the foot and ankle with concomitant osteomyelitis, surgical debridement, combined with systemic or oral antibiotic therapy, may provide the patient with functional limb salvage options. Resection of all grossly infected, necrotic soft tissue and bone should be performed while preserving viable healthy tissues, keeping in mind the potential function of the remaining structures. Staging of procedures is a useful approach in CN of the foot and ankle with concomitant osteomyelitis so that infection is eradicated, leaving healthy viable soft tissue and bone that can maintain definitive long-term correction (**Fig. 2**).

In the presence of large soft tissue or osseous voids, nonbiodegradable cemented antibiotic-impregnated beads and/or spacers can be utilized for eradication of the infection and/or stabilization of joints. Although Buchholz and Engelbrecht first

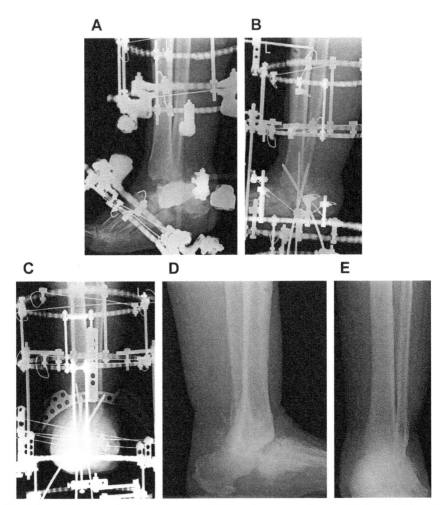

Fig. 2. Lateral lower extremity radiograph (*A*) showing a cemented nonbiodegradable antibiotic spacer after an initial talectomy was performed for the management of a septic diabetic CN of the ankle joint. Lateral (*B*) and anteroposterior (*C*) lower extremity radiographs demonstrating the removal of the cemented nonbiodegradable antibiotic spacer, external fixation modification, and staged tibiocalcaneal arthrodesis 6 weeks after the initial surgery. The external fixator utilized for the arthrodesis site was removed at 12 weeks after the arthrodesis procedure. Final postoperative lateral (*D*) and anteroposterior (*E*) lower extremity radiographs demonstrating the successful limb salvage procedure at 1 year follow-up.

introduced antibiotic-impregnated cement for the treatment of infected hip arthroplasties in 1970, Klemm later utilized a similar technique with gentamicin-impregnated polymethylmethacrylate beads on surgical wire to fill spaces left after debridement of infected bone.[9,10] For over 3 decades, antibiotic-impregnated cement beads and/or spacers have been used in the treatment of osteomyelitis, because this method provides local delivery of concentrated antibiotic(s) while aiming to decrease systemic toxicity. Placement of these antibiotic beads and spacers can also help provide stabilization of the surrounding structures to maintain length and alignment in anticipation of more definitive reconstructive procedures. Recently, external fixation has been reported as a useful adjunct in order to maintain positioning of the foot and ankle with the retained antibiotic beads for the duration of systemic antibiotic therapy. Infectious disease consultation is recommended for many of these clinical case scenarios, because 6 to 8 weeks of parenteral antibiotic therapy may be warranted before proceeding to definitive reconstruction. Once infection has resolved, arthrodesis procedures are the most often cited approaches to provide lasting correction of diabetic CN foot and ankle with concomitant osteomyelitis.[11,12]

Clinical case scenarios of diabetic CN foot and ankle deformities with concomitant osteomyelitis that produce extensive soft tissue loss after surgical debridement require creative strategies for long-term wound closure. The development of negative pressure wound therapy (NPWT) by Morykwas and colleagues[13] has been considered one of the greatest breakthroughs in wound care in the last 30 years. The technique delivers subatmospheric pressure through open-cell foam placed into the wound, ultimately expediting granulation tissue formation and decreasing bacterial counts to promote wound healing. Large wounds in CN and concomitant osteomyelitis may be addressed with NPWT to prepare for final closure using orthobiologic dressings, skin grafts, and/or plastic surgical techniques depending on the wound characteristics. NPWT has also been successfully combined with antibiotic beads and external fixation for treatment of complex soft tissue and bone defects in CN foot and ankle and concomitant osteomyelitis.[14]

SUMMARY

Although a dramatic evolution has occurred for options in the management of diabetic CN of the foot and ankle with concomitant osteomyelitis, studies continue to emphasize the importance of careful patient selection and a multidisciplinary team approach for the overall treatment of these patients. As new research emerges, a better understanding of the pathogenesis and course of these unique coexistent conditions may lead to improved surgical outcomes. Consideration for the future management of the infected Charcot foot and ankle will require further advances in the development of newer classes of antibiotics and improved delivery systems, as the probability of more drug-resistant pathogens is likely to rise.

REFERENCES

1. Chisholm KA, Gilchrist JM. The Charcot joint: a modern neurologic perspective. J Clin Neuromuscul Dis 2011;13:1–13.
2. Sohn MW, Stuck RM, Pinzur M, et al. Lower extremity amputation risk after Charcot arthropathy and diabetic foot ulcer. Diabetes Care 2010;33:98–100.
3. Delmaire M, Maugendre D, Moreno M, et al. Impaired leukocyte function in diabetic patients. Diabet Med 1997;14:29–34.
4. Zgonis T, Stapleton JJ, Shibuya N, et al. Surgically induced Charcot neuroarthropathy following partial forefoot amputation in diabetes. J Wound Care 2007; 16:57–9.
5. Shank CF, Feibel JB. Osteomyelitis in the diabetic foot: diagnosis and management. Foot Ankle Clin 2006;11:775–89.
6. Palestro CJ, Patel M, Freeman SJ, et al. Marrow versus infection in the Charcot joint: indium-111 leukocyte and technetium-99m sulfur colloid scintigraphy. J Nucl Med 1998;39:346–56.
7. Keidar Z, Militianu D, Melamed E, et al. The diabetic foot: initial experience with 18F-FDG PET/CT. J Nucl Med 2005;46:444–9.

8. Ertugrul MB, Baktiroglu S, Salman S, et al. The diagnosis of osteomyelitis of the foot in diabetes: microbiological examination vs. magnetic resonance imaging and labeled leucocyte scanning. Diabet Med 2006;23:649–53.

9. Buchholz H, Engelbrecht H. Depot effects of various antibiotics mixed with Palacos resins. Chirurg 1970;41:511–5.

10. Klemm K. Antibiotic bead chains. Clin Orthop 1993;295:63–76.

11. Stapleton JJ, Zgonis T. Surgical reconstruction of the diabetic Charcot foot: internal, external or combined fixation? Clin Podiatr Med Surg 2012;29:425–33.

12. Pawar A, Dikmen G, Fragomen A, et al. Antibiotic-coated nail for fusion of infected Charcot ankles. Foot Ankle Int 2013;34:80–4.

13. Morykwas MJ, Argenta LC, Shelton-Brown EI, et al. Vacuum-assisted closure: a new method for wound control and treatment: animal studies and basic foundation. Ann Plast Surg 1997;38:553–62.

14. Ramanujam CL, Facaros Z, Zgonis T. Abductor hallucis muscle flap with circular external fixation for Charcot foot osteomyelitis: a case report. Diabet Foot Ankle 2011;2.

Midfoot Crush Injuries

Lawrence A. DiDomenico, DPM, FACFAS[a,b,c,*],
Zachary M. Thomas, DPM[a,b]

KEYWORDS

- Midfoot • Crushing injuries • Tarsometatarsal joint

KEY POINTS

- Treatment of midfoot injuries can be surgical or nonsurgical, depending on the injury, the location, and the extent of the injury.
- Minor injuries usually heal with casting or bracing, whereas more unstable injuries typically need surgery for stability. Whether the injury is in a weight-bearing portion of the foot is also a consideration for surgery.
- It is vitally important that the surgeon makes a detailed assessment of the soft tissues and bones involved with the injury.
- Preservation and maintaining the soft tissue envelope should be of high priority to the surgeon.

INTRODUCTION

Crushing midfoot injuries are a relatively rare occurrence accounting for only 6% of traumatic midfoot injuries.[1,2] Midfoot crush injuries are easily identified but often present a confounding treatment dilemma. Treatment has evolved from reduction and casting to bridge plating, external fixation, and combined pins and screws if accepting.[1] These injuries are often a part of a larger trauma and may be last on a lengthy priority list. In this review, we discuss the anatomy and role of the midfoot and review treatment and associated comorbidities of midfoot crushing injuries.

EPIDEMIOLOGY OF MIDFOOT FRACTURES

In a review of 155 patients at a level 1 trauma center, 72% of fractures were caused in traffic with 52%, 17%, 2.6%, and 1.3% of these traffic injures being caused by car, motorcycle, pedestrian, and bicycle accidents, respectively. Falls accounted for 12% and blast injuries for 8%, and other injuries accounted for the other 8% of midfoot fractures (**Fig. 1**).[3]

Disclosure: None.
[a] Ankle and Foot Care Centers, Youngstown, OH, USA; [b] Heritage Valley Health System, Beaver, PA, USA; [c] Kent State University, College of Podiatric Medicine, Independence, Ohio
* Corresponding author. 8175 Market Street, Youngstown, Ohio 44512.
E-mail address: ld5353@aol.com

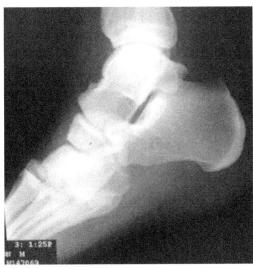

Fig. 1. A 27-year-old man who sustained a significant midfoot injury during a motor vehicle accident.

FUNCTIONAL ANATOMY OF THE MIDFOOT JOINTS

The articulations of the tarsometatarsal joint and midtarsal joint make up the longitudinal arch of the foot. The tarsometatarsal joint consists of 5 metatarsal bases articulating with 3 cuneiforms and the cuboid. The tarsometatarsal joints are bound by 3 groups of ligaments, the plantar, interosseous, and dorsal with the interosseous being stronger than the plantar and the plantar stronger than the dorsal ligaments. The first metatarsal and medial cuneiform make up the medial column, the central 2 metatarsals and their respective intermediate and lateral cuneiforms make up the central column, and the fourth and fifth metatarsals articulating with the cuboid comprise the lateral column. The dorsalis pedis artery and deep peroneal artery course dorsally over the tarsometatarsal joints and are at constant risk for embarrassment during midfoot trauma. The 2 tendons that cause the biggest problems with reduction are the tibialis anterior and peroneus longus, which become incarcerated easily in fracture dislocations of the tarsometatarsal and midtarsal joints. Ouzounian and Shereff,[4] in a landmark study, found that the medial column is relatively stiff and immobile, whereas the lateral column is supple and readily adaptable to changes in terrain with the medial column allowing 3.5 mm of sagittal plane motion, the central column allowing only 0.6 mm of sagittal motion, and the lateral column allowing 13 mm of motion on average. Even though the medial column exhibits less than half the motion of the lateral column, it does provide an important role in gait by transferring force laterally though the tarsometatarsal joint through its available frontal plane motion. Although the second tarsometatarsal joint is known as the keystone, laboratory investigation found that the third tarsometatarsal joint is the joint that bears the greatest load during gait regardless of the foot position or load borne through the complex.[5]

The midtarsal joint complex comprises the talonavicular joint and calcaneocuboid joint. The calcaneocuboid joint contributes relatively little to hindfoot motion; however, the talonavicular articulation contributes to most rearfoot motion.[6] The calcaneocuboid joint is a planar joint that contributes relatively little motion to the hindfoot. This articulation stays relatively stiff so that the cuboid can provide a stable bony alleyway for the peroneus longus to efficiently work. The calcaneocuboid joint must also remain stable so the fourth and fifth metatarsals have a solid foundation with which to articulate with. The talonavicular joint, if damaged by trauma, can result in a staggering loss of pedal adaptive motion.

The navicular comprises 4 articular facets and the site of ligamentous and tendinous attachment. Blood supply to this bone is precarious owning to the large portion of the bone that is covered in articular cartilage. Blood vessels enter on the dorsal and plantar surfaces from the dorsalis pedis and posterior tibial artery via the medial plantar artery, respectively. This bone also receives arterial supply from the insertion of the posterior tibial tendon.[7,8] This arterial pattern leaves the central portion of the navicular in a state of relative avascularity. It is no surprise that stress fractures propagate through the central portion of this bone. The cuboid is a pyramidal-shaped bone with a medial base and lateral apex. The peroneal groove runs along its plantar surface. There are 4 articular facets on the cuboid: distally it articulates with the fourth and fifth metatarsal bases, medially it articulates with the lateral surface of the lateral cuneiform, and proximally the cuboid articulates with the anterior process of the calcaneus. The cuboid is supplied blood by the lateral plantar artery. The talus normally has between 5 and 6 articular surfaces. The talus' blood supply arises from branches of the anterior tibial, posterior tibial, dorsalis pedis, and peroneal arteries.[9]

THE SOFT TISSUE ENVELOPE

Treatments of midfoot injuries in which soft tissues have been mismanaged or neglected have resulted in poor outcomes. The foot has a thin soft tissue layer covering a complex network of muscle, tendon, ligaments, neurovascular structures, and bony architecture. The soft tissue envelope is important not only for wound coverage but for the vascularity of the local tissue and bone. With respect to trauma, the basic principles followed by the Arbeitsgemeinschaft für Osteosynthesefragen group included anatomic reduction and stable internal fixation. Careful attention to soft tissue handling and functional rehabilitation of the injured site is vital for posttraumatic management. Functional rehabilitation involves restoring muscular power and normal or as close to normal biomechanics.

The soft tissue envelope has been recognized as the vascular envelope responsible for fostering the healing of the injury. The importance of surgical anatomy and atraumatic techniques can prevent devascularization and prevent adverse surgical sequelae after an injury. Proper soft tissue handling is mandatory as is the use of proper tools such as fine skin hooks that permit the manipulation of the skin and soft tissues without further damage.

A logical method of reconstruction of the soft tissues is necessary to allow bone to heal and limb to function well. These principles remain in the acute or chronic conditions with or without fractures involving the soft tissue. It is vitally important for the treating surgeon understand the approach and use of soft tissue techniques relative to the soft tissues in these complex injuries. Understanding the appropriate time to operate and the relationship between the soft tissue and the bone is key in the management of these multifaceted injuries. Fracture blisters should be resolved before starting surgical care. Examining the patient for posttraumatic edema reduction is necessary before surgical intervention. A simple inexpensive examination is the wrinkle test. When skin lines are present, this is a good indication that surgical care can be provided with a more predictable outcome of the soft tissue envelope.

COMPARTMENT SYNDROME

The foot comprises several myofascial compartments. There is disagreement as to the exact number, but for completeness this discussion we will refer to 10 separate compartments. These compartments are the medial, calcaneal, superficial (plantar), lateral, 4 interosseous, adductor, and dorsal (**Box 1**).

The pathophysiology of compartment syndrome is an increase in interstitial pressure with a decrease in capillary blood flow, which leads to a decrease in perfusion pressure and subsequent inadequate tissue blood perfusion. Compartment syndrome can occur up to 36 hours after insult. At 4 hours, muscle begins to necrose and only has an 8- to 10-hour window of viability; after this time has passed, the risk of infection outweighs any potential benefits of decompression.[10] Fulkerson and colleagues,[11] in a review, contended that muscle begins to lose viability at 2 hours, and at 8 hours 90% of muscle shows injury, but it takes 12 hours to produce permanent contracture. They also stated that neural deficits begin at 30 minutes and are irreversible from 12 to 24 hours after injury, depending on the patient, if treatment is not instituted. With this time table, it is obvious that once neural symptoms set in, the clock begins ticking rapidly to institute treatment in the form of fasciotomy. Compartment syndrome occurs in 2% to 12% of all lower-extremity trauma, with 69% of cases resulting from fracture. In a case series of 12 patients by Manoli and colleagues[12], 3 were a result of multiple metatarsal fractures. Diagnosis has historically been made clinically by the "5 P's": pain, paresthesia, pulselessness, pallor, and paralysis; however, at this time, pain and paresthesia have been the only 2 clinical symptoms of diagnostic value.[13] Definitive diagnosis is made by wick catheter readings of 30 mm Hg or higher. This number is derived from the forearm and leg, which has led others to use the range of 10 to 30 mm hg below diastolic blood pressure for diagnosis[11] Phillips and colleagues[14] also found a tuning fork is sensitive at 35 to 40 mm Hg. Shuler and colleagues[15] in 2010 found normalized near-infrared spectroscopy to be useful in diagnosis in compartment syndrome. However the diagnosis is made, treatment must not be delayed. Before any bone work can be done, the tissues must be addressed. Several fasciotomy techniques have been described over the years, but for our purposes we describe the single medial and dorsal approach. From the medial approach, all compartments may be accessed except for the interosseous and adductor, which are approached by 2 dorsal linear incisions. Once decompression is achieved for massive midfoot injuries, an external fixator is an appropriate adjunct to stabilize the bony segments. Osseous stability is a key prerequisite for tissue viability. Once the tissues display viability, definitive internal fixation may be attempted. Typically, decompression of the fascial compartments is prophylactic for fracture blisters (**Figs. 2–4**).

Box 1
Myofascial compartments of the foot

- *Medial compartment:* flexor hallucis brevis, abductor hallucis
- *Calcaneal compartment:* quadratus plantae
- *Superficial compartment:* flexor digitorum brevis, flexor digitorum longus, lumbricales
- *Lateral compartment:* abductor digiti minimi, flexor digiti quiniti
- *Interosseous compartment*[4]: respective dorsal and plantar interosseous
- *Adductor compartment:* adductor hallucis
- *Dorsal compartment:* Extensor digitorum Brevis, Dorsal Extrinsic Muscle tendons

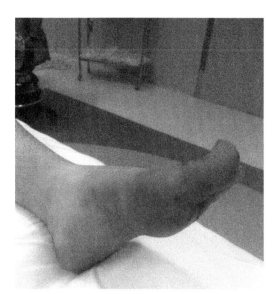

Fig. 2. Preoperative view of a 33-year-old man who experienced a forefoot and midfoot crush injury with a compartment syndrome (12,000 pounds crushed his foot). Surprisingly, there were no fractures to his injured extremity.

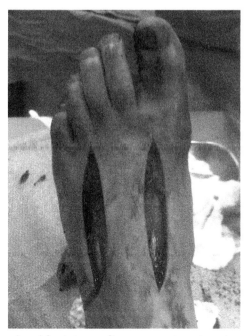

Fig. 3. Post–2-incision dorsal fasciotomy after a compartment syndrome to the foot.

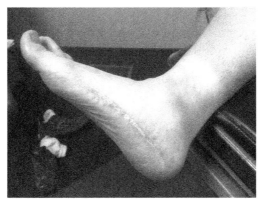

Fig. 4. Patient who underwent a single medial fasciotomy 2 years earlier.

FRACTURE BLISTERS

Fracture blisters occur after the soft tissues have undergone various degrees of insult. Historically thought of as only presenting with high-energy injuries, reports show these blisters occurring in injuries as innocuous as occurring from 4-foot falls.[16] The pathogenesis of fracture blisters is multifactorial; shear or torqueing force results in separation of the stratified squamous cell layer from the underlying vascular dermal layer by inflowing edema fluid. As this occurs, a relative tissue hypoxia results from vasodilatation, edema, and increasing interstitial pressure, which results in separation of the epidermis from the dermis. The level of separation differentiates fluid-filled blisters from hemorrhagic blisters. Fluid-filled blisters are tense and clear. They result from partial separation of the epidermis from the dermis with residual epidermal cells remaining on the surface of the dermis. Hemorrhagic blisters present as flaccid and blood filled. The blisters result from a complete epidermal-dermal separation (source). The timing of these blisters is anywhere from 12 hours to 3 weeks after trauma.[17,18] Prophylactic measures include elevation, ice, compression, and early bony stabilization.[16] Treatment protocols are less definitive. In several reports spanning 12 years, it has been stated consistently that there are no universal guidelines for treatment of associated fracture blisters when treating fractures.[16,18–20] Suggested protocols include incision and drainage with roof left in place as biologic dressing, silvadene cream of betadine paint and compressive dressing applied, and surgical intervention delayed because of the presence of skin lines and blister epithelization. Others include deroofing all blisters and treat with silvadene twice daily until epithelization. Also, investigators have advocated leaving blisters intact until skin lines return and deroofing at the time of surgery and paint with betadine. Some investigators suggest that fracture blisters be treated with the same algorithms as second-degree burns.[16,18–20] Whatever the treatment may be, the consensus among reports seems to be that incisions must be placed through supple, epithelialized tissue. It is idealistic to think that every massive midfoot injury that presents should be stabilized in time to avoid fracture blisters; however, this has proven untrue many times over. Again, external fixation plays a pivotal role in the treatment of the mangled midfoot in the presence of fracture blisters. Whether it is circular fixation with skinny wires and pins or delta frame, these devices allow the bony segments to be stabilized while granting access to the soft tissues for constant monitoring and management until a time that definite management can be attempted. In some cases, the external fixator may be the definitive method of fixation (**Fig. 5**).

TARSOMETATARSAL JOINT CRUSH INJURIES

This subset of injuries to Lisfranc joint differs from midfoot sprain in that crushing injuries to the tarsometatarsal joint do not follow the exact mechanism of injury as ligamentous Lisfranc injuries. Ligamentous Lisfranc injuries follow a twisting injury, whereas a crushing injury tends to be a more direct pattern that includes axial loading; projectile, blunt, or penetrating trauma by foreign object; or blast injury. Outcomes related to Lisfranc joint crush injuries are unfavorable. There is a 25% rate of posttraumatic arthritis in Lisfranc joint injuries regardless of age or gender.[21–23] In a study of patients with high-energy open Lisfranc trauma, Nithyananth and colleagues[24] found 5 deaths and 1 amputation, and of the 16 remaining patients there was a 77% spontaneous fusion rate. These investigators used open fracture protocols with multiple debridements and multiple k-wire fixation. In the small bones of the foot, k-wires can navigate small, comminuted areas in which screw fixation cannot. This is also true for skinny wires in circular external fixation with or without the use of olives for fracture reduction. The bones of the midfoot are largely cancellous and the risk for impaction, shortening, and rotational deformities are high. Aggressive bone grafting at the time of surgery is warranted in these cases. In crushing injuries to small articulating segments in the foot in which bone grafting is being used, interfragmentary compression is not necessary and can cause additional deformity. Positional screws, neutralization, and buttress plating is the method of choice in fixation of these injuries if feasible. Many of these injuries will show significant cartilage blowout and require primary arthrodesis. Temporary external fixation may be needed if significant comminution and instability are present. Multiple other surgeries may be needed first for life-threatening injuries or if the patient presents late and the soft tissues are not fit for open surgery. In patients who are not candidates for open surgery, this may be definitive fixation. The first second, and third tarsometatarsal joints are considered nonessential and may be fused with relatively low morbidity, the fourth and fifth tarsometatarsal

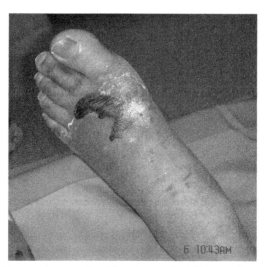

Fig. 5. A 38-year-old man who sustained forefoot and midfoot crush injury. Note the post-traumatic edema and fracture blister.

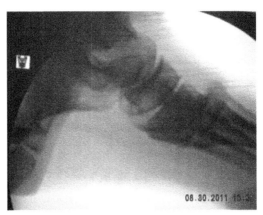

Fig. 6. A 45-year-old woman with a dorsal crush injury. Note the instability at Lisfranc and the mid foot.

joints play a significant role in adapting to terrain and, if destroyed, may cause long-term stiffness and difficulty ambulating. Attempts to salvage these joints should be made; however, in crushing injuries, the energy of injury may dictate the decision (**Figs. 6–9**).

CHOPART JOINT TRAUMA

The talonavicular and calcaneocuboid joint make up the Chopart joint. The talonavicular joint accounts for most rearfoot motion with 36.7° ± 13° of motion. The calcaneocuboid joint only exhibits 14.4° ± 6° of motion. In a study of simulated arthrodesis of the triple joint complex, Astion and coworkers[6] found that by fusing the talonavicular joint, the subtalar and calcaneocuboid joints' ranges of motion decreased to 2° and that the posterior tibial tendon excursion decreased to 25% of its original value.[6] Trauma to the talonavicular joint of any kind can result in deleterious changes to pedal motion. Every attempt at salvaging this joint should be undertaken before primary arthrodesis is considered. However, as with every crushing injury, the energy of the

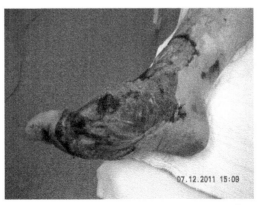

Fig. 7. A 33-year-old man who experienced a degloving along with fracture and dislocation injury after a crush injury from a motorcycle accident. This patient underwent multiple debridements, negative pressure therapy, hyperbaric oxygen treatment, percutaneous pinning and a split thickness skin graft.

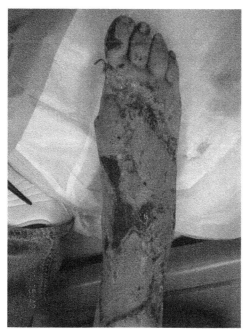

Fig. 8. A 33-year-old man who experienced a degloving along with fracture and dislocation injury after a crush injury from a motorcycle accident. This patient underwent multiple debridements, negative pressure therapy, hyperbaric oxygen treatment, percutaneous pinning and a split thickness skin graft.

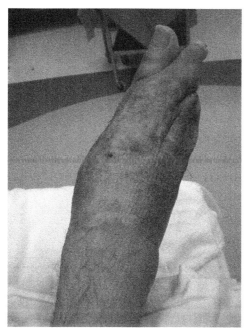

Fig. 9. A patient presented with postoperative crush injury requesting reconstruction of the injured foot. This patient experienced partial loss after a crush injury.

injury will dictate treatment algorithms. The talus and navicular's precarious blood supply has been illustrated previously in this report. If this joint sustains severe comminution, primary arthrodesis should be considered. Importance of position in fusion of the talonavicular joint cannot be stressed enough. The posterior tibial tendon, saphenous nerve and vein, and the spring ligament may all be traumatized or incarcerated. Careful handling of the soft tissues is necessary. In this area, mono- or mini-rail external fixation may be needed to keep the talonavicular joint out to length while bone graft incorporating. If there is an associated talar neck fracture, the fixation must either span the entire site or hold the talonavicular joint to length while the talar neck and head are reconstructed. Buttress plating with multiple wires may be used as well to disperse forces across the graft site and to provide stability to the healing soft tissues. Fully threaded positional screws may be used as well (**Figs. 10** and **11**).

NAVICULAR COMMINUTION

The mechanism of action of comminuted navicular fractures tends to be a direct blow from an outside force such as a projectile object, axial loading injury, or blast.[25] If the injury is open, open fracture protocols should be instituted. Because the navicular's proximal and distal surfaces are covered with articular cartilage, most of these injuries have at least some intra-articular involvement. Although considered a nonessential joint, arthrosis of the naviculocuneiform joints can lead to chronic midfoot pain. Intra-articular damage to the talonavicular joint can have significant functional consequences. Comminution of the navicular can lead to loss of mechanical advantage of the posterior tibial tendon and frank collapse of the medial column. The mainstay of acute navicular crushing injuries is reduction with bridging external fixation to keep the midfoot out to length. If the soft tissues allow, acute treatment entails early open

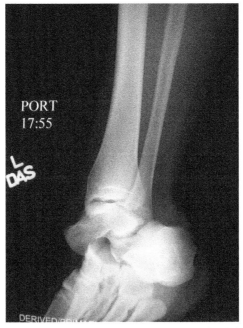

Fig. 10. Prereduction radiograph shows an isolated talar navicular dislocation after a motor vehicle accident.

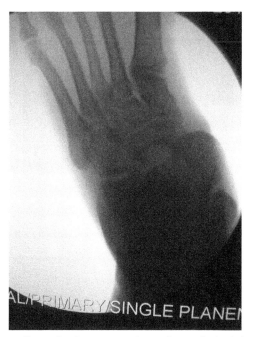

Fig. 11. Prereduction radiographs show a complete talar navicular joint dislocation.

reduction and internal fixation with screws, k-wires, and bridge plating if necessary from the talus to the first metatarsal, which can be removed once consolidation has ocurred.[2] Bone grafting plays a key role in comminuted navicular fractures because of the potential for significant bone loss during trauma. External fixation is used to stabilize the medial column and allow for incorporation of the bone graft and fixated native fragments. For isolated navicular comminution, a mono- or minirail is used. The rail fixator pins are placed distally in the medial cuneiform and first metatarsal and proximally in the talus or calcaneus. Often, 2 mono-rail fixators are needed to provide uniform diastasis. The second fixator is placed laterally into the calcaneus and cuboid or fifth metatarsal. Navicular comminution and gross midfoot comminution may be better suited for a delta frame with pins placed appropriately in the tibia, mid-foot, and hindfoot.[26] If a ring fixator is chosen, it should be used with olive wires running transversely through the metatarsal parabola and the rearfoot complex to provide stable distraction. As stated earlier, the navicular is largely covered in articular cartilage. This factor is important when comminution destroys part or all of the articulating surfaces. Conservative treatment for posttraumatic midfoot arthritis begins with bracing and physical therapy. If conservative measures fail, surgical intervention is warranted. Naviculocuneiform fusion will not affect pedal mechanics significantly; however, fusion of the talonavicular joint can greatly alter the mechanics of the patient's gait. In cases of total articular blowout a talonavicular-cuneiform fusion will gather sufficient bone for solid union and ultimate freedom in position of fusion (**Fig. 12**).

ISOLATED CUBOID COMMINUTION

The literature lacks reports dealing with cuboid fractures. This lack of reports is directly proportional to the incidence of cuboid fractures as a whole. In the United Kingdom, there is an incidence of 1.8 per 10,000 annually.[27] Crushing injuries of the cuboid, to no surprise,

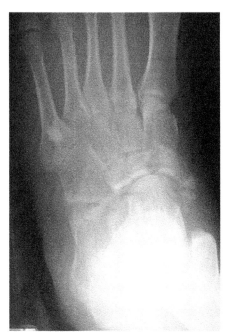

Fig. 12. A preoperative radiograph demonstrating a displace fracture of the navicular prior to open reduction and internal fixation.

are rarely reported in the literature. This injury occurs from direct blow/blast or from forced abduction in the "Nutcracker" injury pattern mechanism. Direct blowing injuries to the cuboid occur from a direct strike of a foreign object, such as blunt trauma or penetrating open trauma. If the fracture is open, open fracture protocol should be instituted. With indirect injury mechanisms, the comminuted cuboid fracture is a component of a larger injury pattern. The forced abduction causes navicular subluxation, avulsion fracture, and crushing of the cuboid[1] and is often associated with a second metatarsal fracture. Historical treatment algorithms have given way to advances in internal and external fixation. In the late 1960s Dewar and Evans[28] recommended primary calcaneocuboid joint fusion, Main and Jowlett[1] and Ebizie[29] advocated plaster casting and triple arthrodesis for late arthritic symptoms. Treatment decision making begins with x-ray and often computed tomography scan findings. With a crushing injury to the cuboid, there will invariably be shortening to the lateral column, which can lead to a painful flatfoot deformity.[30] If there is displacement found, ORIF with bone grafting should be attempted. Depending on the severity of comminution, surgical intervention may entail simple open reduction and internal fixation with or without bone grafting and pins or screws to bridge plating for more cavernous defects needing to be grafted. Again, depending on the level of lateral column collapse and stability, an external fixator may be needed to hold the lateral column out to length. Whatever the intervention chosen, attention must be directed to the peroneus longus and its sulcus on the plantar surface of the cuboid. All attempts should be made to preserve the gliding motion of this osseo-tendinous unit (**Fig. 13**).[26,30,31]

GLOBAL MIDFOOT CRUSHING

These injuries often are part of a polytrauma case. When gross instability to the midfoot, is present, early stabilization with external fixation allows the soft tissues to settle before

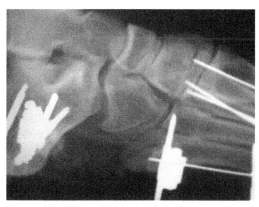

Fig. 13. A lateral radiograph shows an isolated cuboid fracture in a case in which external fixation has been applied to maintain the length while the soft tissues recover from the crush injury.

more definitive fixation with bone grafting can be instituted. In fracture patterns that have no primary cortical bone contact, tricortical structural bone grafting should be used. The same principles stated previously can be relied on for definitive management; however, with global comminution, most injuries warrant primary fusion (**Table 1**).

REHABILITATION

The period of treatment for a midfoot fracture is directly related to the location and type of fracture and the time of immobilization. The goal of rehabilitation should

Table 1
Proposed classification system for bone grafting

Graft Site Type	Graft Technique	Primary Graft Indication	Secondary Graft Indication	Internal Fixation
Complete cortical apposition	Shear-strain relieving	Cancellous autograft	Cancellous allograft	Screw: Compression Plating: Locked or nonlocking
Partial cortical apposition	Cancellous backfilling	Cancellous autograft	Cancellous allograft	Screw: Positional or compression Plating: Combination locking/ nonlocking
Bony gap <2 cm	Tricortical corticocancellous graft	Tricortical calcaneal, Tricortical iliac crest	Tricortical allograft of choice	Screw: Positional Plate: Combination locking/ nonlocking
Bony gap >2 cm	Cortical strut + cancellous backfilling	Fibular strut or iliac crest + mixture autograft/ allograft cancellous	Banked corticocancellous graft	Screw: Positional Plate: Combination locking nonlocking

emphasize restoring full range of motion, strength, proprioception, and endurance while attempting to maintain independence. Continuation of preinjury activity level is the goal with this patient population. To provide patients a pathway to rehabilitation, the local fracture/injury must be stable from the operative or nonoperative management.

The goal of rehabilitation is to return the full function with a painless, plantigrade foot. Some midfoot injuries may not hinder activities of daily living but may obstruct the individual's ability to work because of pain and restricted weight bearing. Gait training using appropriate assistive devices can help individuals with ambulation and allow them to move about independently. When indicated, the patient may progressively increase range of motion and proprioceptive and strengthening exercises until a normal gait and full function is evident. Orthotics or ankle foot orthosis may be indicated in some cases to protect the foot, relieve discomfort, and promote a functional gait pattern.

Displaced fractures will require surgery. These patients will typically require no weight bearing for several months followed by rehabilitation. Therapy and range of motion exercises are not started until bony union/stability has occurred. Bone healing may occur within 6 to 12 weeks, but bone strength and the ability of the bone to sustain a heavy load may take up to several months to years to return. Once healing has occurred, the individual may resume full activities of daily living. It is important to educate the patient not to overload the fracture site until the bone has regained its full strength.

SUMMARY

Treatment of midfoot injuries is surgical or nonsurgical, depending on the injury, the location, and the extent of the injury. Minor injuries usually heal with casting or bracing, whereas more unstable injuries typically need surgery for stability. Whether the injury is in a weight-bearing portion of the foot is also a consideration for surgery.

It is vitally important that the surgeon makes a detailed assessment of the soft tissues and bones involved with the injury. Preservation and maintaining the soft tissue envelope should be of high priority to the surgeon. Loss of bone in the midfoot can drastically shorten the foot. Keeping the columns out to length is key in the immediate postoperative timeframe for favorable long-term results. Surgical decisions should be based on issues such as the condition of the soft tissue and if there was any loss of bone in the fracture, how big the gap is in the dislocation or fracture, and if there is any instability in the foot. Nonsurgical treatment may be done if there is no loss of bone length, and if the gap is less than 2 mm. Treatment in this case would be casting for about 4 to 6 weeks. If surgery is performed, the patient will not be able to bear weight for at least 4 weeks.

The authors conclude that the importance of treating midfoot injuries adequately is shown in how the midfoot is needed for function with weight bearing and its relationship between the front and the back of the foot. It is also important to ensure that the patient is able to ambulate with a normal gait or as close to normal as possible.

REFERENCES

1. Main BJ, Jowett RL. Injuries of the midtarsal joint. J Bone Joint Surg Br 1975; 57(1):89–97.
2. Makawana NK, Liefland MR. Injuries of the midfoot. Curr Orthop 2005;19:231–42.
3. Richter M, Wippermann B, Krettek C, et al. Fractures and fracture dislocations of the midfoot: occurrence, cause and long-term results. Foot Ankle Int 2001;22(5):392–8.

4. Ouzounian TJ, Shereff MJ. In vitro determination of midfoot motion. Foot Ankle 1989;10:140–6.
5. Lakin RC, DeGnore LT, Pienkowski D. Contact mechanics of normal tarsometatarsal joints. J Bone Joint Surg Am 2001;83(4):520–8.
6. Astion DJ, Deland JT, Otis JC, et al. Motion of the hindfoot after simulated arthrodesis. J Bone Joint Surg Am 1997;79(2):241–6.
7. Kelikian AS. Chapter 2 Sarrafian's anatomy of the foot and ankle. 3rd edition. Philadelphia: Lippincott Williams and Wilkins; 2011.
8. Lee S, Anderson RB. Stress fractures of the tarsal navicular. Foot Ankle Clin N Am 2004;9:85–104.
9. Kelikian AS. Chapter 7 Sarrafian's anatomy of the foot and ankle. 3rd edition. Philadelphia: Lippincott Williams and Wilkins; 2011.
10. Perry MD, Manoli A. Foot compartment syndrome. Orthop Clin North Am 2001; 32(1):103–11.
11. Fulkerson E, Razi A, Tejwani N. Review: acute compartment syndrome of the foot. Foot Ankle Int 2003;24(2):180–7.
12. Manoli A II, Anton JF. Acute Foot Compartment Syndromes. Journal of Orthopaedic Trauma 1992;6(2):223–8.
13. Myerson M. Diagnosis and treatment of compartment syndrome of the foot. Orthopedics 1990;13(7):711–7.
14. Phillips JH, Mackinnon SE, Beatty SE, et al. Vibratory sensory testing in acute compartment syndromes: a clinical and experimental study. Plast Reconstr Surg 1987;79(5):796–801.
15. Shuler MS, Reisman WM, Kinsey TL, et al. Correlation between muscle oxygenation and compartment pressures in acute compartment syndrome in the leg. J Bone Joint Surg Am 2010;92(4):863–70.
16. Wallace GF, Sullivan J. Fracture blisters. Clin Podiatr Med Surg 1995;12:801–12.
17. Varela CD, Vaughan TK, Carr JB, et al. Fracture blisters. Clinical and pathological aspects. J Orthop Trauma 1993;7:417–27.
18. Ballo F, Maroon M, Millon SJ. Fracture blisters. J Am Acad Dermatol 1994;30: 1033–4.
19. Giordano CP, Koval KJ. Treatment of fracture blisters: a prospective study of 53 cases. J Orthop Trauma 1995;9:171–6.
20. Strauss EJ, Petrucelli G, Bong M, et al. Blisters associated with lower extremity fractures: results of a prospective treatment protocol. J Orthop Trauma 2006; 20:618–22.
21. Kuo RS, Tejwani NC, DiGiovanni CW, et al. Outcome after open reduction and internal fixation of Lisfranc joint injuries. J Bone Joint Surg Am 2000;82-A(11):1009–10.
22. Resch S, Stenstrom A. The treatment of tarsometatarsal injuries. Foot Ankle Int 1990;11(3):117–23.
23. Herscovici D, Scaduto JM. Management of high-energy foot and ankle injuries in the geriatric population. Geriatr Orthop Surg Rehabil 2012;3(1):33–44.
24. Nithyananth M, Boopalan PR, Titus VT, et al. Long-term outcome of high-energy open lisfranc injuries: a retrospective study. J Trauma 2011;70(3):710–6.
25. DiGiovanni CW. Fractures of the navicular. Foot Ankle Clin N Am 2004;9:25–63.
26. Ballmer FT, Hertel PM, Ballmer RPJ. Othter applications of the small AO external fixator to the lower limb. Injury 1994;25(Suppl 4):S-D69–76.
27. Court-Brown CM, Zinna S, Ekrol I. Classification and epidemiology of midfoot fractures. Foot 2006;16(3):138–41.
28. Dewar FP, Evans DC. Occult fracture subluxation of the mid-tarsal joint. J Bone Joint Surg 1968;50B:386.

29. Ebizie AO. Crush fractures of the cuboid from indirect violence. Injury 1991;22(5): 414–6.
30. Mihalich RM, Early JS. Management of cuboid crush injuries. Foot Ankle Clin N Am 2006;11:121–6.
31. Swords MP, Schramski M, Switzer K, et al. Chopart fractures and dislocations. Foot Ankle Clin N Am 2008;13:679–93.

Fractures of the Talus

Yury Bykov, MD

KEYWORDS

• Talus • Hindfoot • Tarsal • Fractures • Trauma

KEY POINTS

- Fractures of the talus are relatively rare injuries that usually occur as the result of high-energy trauma.
- The entire patient needs to be assessed, and more life-threatening injuries need to take priority.
- The soft tissue envelope around the hindfoot is tenuous and must be protected. At times, that may require emergent surgery to reduce and stabilize the bony deformity that is compromising the skin.

INTRODUCTION

The talus is the most proximal bone of the hindfoot that couples the foot to the leg. It is the second most common fracture of the tarsal bones, second in frequency to the calcaneous. However, overall injuries to the talus are relatively rare, and most surgeons have little experience in managing them. This article discusses fractures of the talus, including injuries to the talar neck, body, head, and processes. Although subtalar dislocations and osteochondral injuries are important topics, they are not addressed in this article.

The focus of this article will include:

Bony and vascular anatomy
Initial history/physical and radiographic assessment
Timing of surgery
Surgical approaches
Methods of fixation
Postoperative care
Outcomes and complication
Salvage and reconstructive procedures

Disclosure: None.
Orthopaedic Surgery, VSAS Orthopaedics, Lehigh Valley Hospital, 1250 South Cedar Crest Boulevard, Suite 110, Allentown, PA 18103, USA
E-mail address: yubykov@hotmail.com

Clin Podiatr Med Surg 31 (2014) 509–521
http://dx.doi.org/10.1016/j.cpm.2014.06.004
0891-8422/14/$ – see front matter © 2014 Elsevier Inc. All rights reserved.

ANATOMY
Bony Anatomy

The talus is the connection between the ankle joint and the foot, with 60% of it being covered by cartilage. There are no muscular origins or insertions into the talus. Most authors break up bony anatomy of the talus into distinct anatomic regions: body, neck, head, lateral process, and posterior process.

The body of the talus is a large trapezoidal shaped dome. It is wider anteriorly than posteriorly. It has a convex superior surface to articulate with the weight-bearing plafond of the distal tibia. Medially and laterally it has cartilaginous surfaces that articulate with medial and lateral malleoli. Inferiorly, it has a concave articular surface that articulates with the posterior facet of the calcaneous.

The head of the talus is a convex round surface that articulates with the navicular bone distally and with the calcaneous plantarly through anterior and middle facets.

The neck connects the head to the body. It bears no articular surface. It originates from the medial side of the body and angles both plantarly and medially.

The lateral process originates from the lateral side of the body. Laterally and superiorly it has a cartilaginous surface that articulates with the distal fibula. Plantarly and medially it articulates with posterior facet of the calcaneous.

The posterior process is separated by the grove of flexor hallucis longus. It is covered by articular cartilage superiorly to articulate with distal tibia and plantarly to articulate with the posterior facet of the calcaneous.

Vascular Supply

All 3 distal arteries—posterior tibial, dorsalis pedis (anterior tibial), and peroneal artery—provide vascularity to the talus.[1]

The posterior tibial artery gives off a branch to the deltoid ligament and the artery of the tarsal canal. It is the most important supply to the talar dome. It is usually the last blood supply left remaining in type III Hawkins talar neck fractures. The deltoid ligament needs to be protected during surgery to preserve it.

The anterior tibial artery provides blood supply to the talar head and neck via the dorsalis pedis artery.

The perforation peroneal artery gives off artery of the tarsal sinus. Along with the artery of the tarsal canal, they form a vascular sling over the inferior talar neck; both provide supply to the talar dome.

There are extensive intraosseous anastomoses among the 3 arteries. It is potentially possible to restore blood flow to the talus if 1 of the 3 arteries remains undamaged.

INITIAL ASSESSMENT

Fractures of the talus are typically high-energy injuries, often seen after a motor vehicle accident or a fall from a great height. A thorough history and physical examination of the patient must be performed. Because these injuries occur in high-energy trauma, often the patient may have other injuries that need to be assessed and addressed. When appropriate, a full advanced trauma life support (ATLS) protocol needs to be performed, and life-threatening injuries should be addressed.

Injury to the talus is usually suspected when pain, swelling, and bruising at the ankle present, prompting initial radiographs. Typically an anteriorposterior (AP) and a lateral views of the ankle would be obtained in an emergency room setting. Once injury to the talus is diagnosed or suspected, more dedicated radiographic imaging should be obtained.

Radiographs

Three views of the ankle (AP, mortise, and the lateral views), AP view of the foot, and a Canale view should be obtained. Often radiographs obtained in an emergency setting are of marginal quality. The diagnostic value of the radiographs diminishes as the quality of radiographic imaging deteriorates. One must insist on proper radiographs to make appropriate decisions.

AP and mortise views allows visualization of the lateral process as well as the talar dome, particularly osteochondral injuries and body fractures in the sagittal plane. Depending on the specific plane of the fracture, it may be more visible in either of these views.

A lateral view of the ankle allows good visualization of the talar neck fractures. On a good lateral view, there will be a single shadow of the superior convexity of the talar body, meaning the lateral and the medial sides of the talar dome are collinear. This view allows the visualization of tibiotalar articulation, subtalar articulation, and talar navicular articulation. Dislocation or subluxations in any of these joints can usually be diagnosed on this view.

AP of the foot allows visualization of the talonavicular joint in that plane. It will allow visualization of the fracture of the talar head. Most talar neck fractures will not be well visualized on this view.

The Canale view is the special view to assess the talar neck. This would be difficult to obtain in emergency settings. This can be obtained in the office setting, as well as operating room fluoroscopically, to assess intraoperative reduction.

This view is obtained by taking an image 75° from the plantar surface of the foot and either pronation of the foot 15° or more commonly rolling the C-arm 15° from AP plane toward the medial side.

Although the lateral view visualizes displacement and angulation in the sagittal plane (flexion/extension), the Canale view allows for assessment of the neck in the coronal plane (valgus/varus). The presence of comminution, usually medially, can also often be assessed on this view.

Advanced Imaging

Computed tomography (CT) allows visualization of small osteochondral fractures, particularly involving the talar dome as well as subtalar and talonavicular joints. It also allows for an appreciation of the amount of comminution that may be encountered intraoperatively. Although not mandatory for all fractures, it is this author's preference to obtain a CT on all injuries of the talus for operative planning.

Magnetic resonance imaging (MRI) is rarely obtained. When it is obtained, it is done incidentally in a patient who has pain, swelling, and inability to bear weight, but otherwise normal initial radiographic imaging to make a diagnosis. Some authors have used MRI to monitor for presence of avascular necrosis (AVN) in the postoperative period.

Bone scan is also rarely obtained. It can occasionally be used to diagnose a stress injury. It has no obvious utility in a trauma setting.

INITIAL MANAGEMENT AND TIMING

Historically, all of these injuries were considered emergencies, and reduction with internal fixation needed to be performed promptly to avoid AVN. Most authors now agree that the AVN occurs as the result of initial injury rather than timing of the internal fixation. Therefore, the timing of surgery is focused more on the condition of soft tissue envelope.

Injuries in which the soft tissue envelope is compromised by bony displacement and deformity require urgent treatment to avoid soft tissue necrosis. These injuries place the limb in jeopardy. This may often require a trip to the operating room for closed or open reduction with placement of temporary external fixator or temporary K-wire. If closed reduction is not possible or satisfactory, one must be ready to perform open reduction with temporary or permanent hardware to preserve the tenuous soft tissue envelope.

In cases in which there is no threat to the soft tissue from bony deformity, it is most prudent to wait for the swelling to improve before undertaking open reduction with internal fixation. The patient is placed in a well padded splint and encouraged to elevate the extremity above the level of the heart. Some authors use cryotherapy and pneumatic compression devices for comfort and to eliminate the swelling. When there is evidence of wrinkling of the skin, surgery should be safe to perform.

As stated previously, these injuries often occur in a multitraumatized patient, and other life-threatening injuries must be taken under consideration when timing surgery.

MANAGEMENT OF SPECIFIC FRACTURES
Talar Neck

These fractures can be classified by Hawkins into grades I, II, and III[2]:

    Grade I nondisplaced fracture
    Grade II fracture with dislocation of subtalar joint
    Grade III fracture with dislocation of subtalar and ankle joint

Kelly and Canale later described a grade IV fracture[3] with dislocation of subtalar, ankle, and talonavicular joints.

Nonoperative care must be considered with great caution for these injuries. Only truly nondisplaced fractures can be managed nonoperatively. Minimally displaced fractures usually require operative care. The author recommends nonoperative care in the fracture that can only be seen on MRI or fractures that are seen with difficulty on CT. Fractures that are obviously visible on radiograph are probably not truly nondisplaced and in most healthy patients should be treated operatively after an informed discussion. If one is considering nonoperative care based on plain radiographic images, a CT should be seriously considered to confirm lack of displacement. A little more leeway can be given to patients with limited or no mobility at baseline or neuropathy, as well as patients with poor soft tissue envelope because of peripheral vascular disease or burns to the surgical site. A good rule to follow is to operatively stabilize if doubt exists.

Nonoperative care consists of splinting or casting in slight equinus. Equinus position for talar neck fractures is preferred, because these fractures are believed to be dorsiflexion injuries. The patients are converted to neutral position around 4 weeks. Range of motion is started at around 6 to 8 weeks. Weight bearing is avoided for about 10 to 12 weeks. Frequent radiographic follow-up is mandatory in the office on a weekly or biweekly bases for the first 4 weeks. If there is a concern about displacement, serious consideration must be given regarding switching to operative care.

Percutaneous stabilization is rarely performed. It consists of placement of percutaneous screws in either retrograde or antegrade directions.

Indications for percutaneous stabilization include:

1. Nondisplaced fractures in a patient who is going to the operating room for other procedures

2. Fractures in patients with limited mobility, neuropathy, vascular insufficiency, or other conditions in which there is a relative contraindication to making an incision or under conditions in which a reasonable closed reduction can be obtained. One must use clinical judgment of what is reasonable. Clearly, a reduction that is reasonable in an 85-year-old nursing home patient may be unreasonable in a 20 year old athlete
3. Patients with nondisplaced isolated fractures may choose to undergo percutaneous stabilization after discussion of risks and benefits; the benefit of performing percutaneous stabilization in these patients ensures that displacement does not occur and allows earlier mobilization of foot and ankle

Technique

A screw can be placed ether antegrade from posterior lateral direction interval between peroneal and flexor hallucis longus tendons. Because the talar neck is medially deviated from talar body, one needs to aim in that direction when placing the antegrade screw. The great toe is a good landmark to aim toward. Medial percutaneous screws in the antegrade direction cannot be safely performed due to the posteriormedial neurovascular bundle. Retrograde screws are placed from the talar head into the body from either medial or lateral sides. The talonavicular joint often needs to be subluxed to allow for placement of the retrograde screws. Regardless of how these screws are placed, the heads of these screws need to be well countersunk to avoid intra-articular irritation. Alternatively, headless screws may be used.

Closed reduction when needed is achieved by axial traction and plantar flexion. The Canale view should be used to assess for coronal plane reduction, and the foot should be deviated medially or laterally to achieve proper reduction. K-wires are used for provisional fixation. Definitive hardware is placed once the reduction is satisfactory. If closed reduction is short of anatomic, one must consider conversion to an open procedure. This can also be used for injuries in which the skin is compromised by bony deformity. In that scenario, the fracture does not have to be anatomic, but rather it is placed in an alignment in which the soft tissue envelope is not threatened. The length of the talar neck and height of the hindfoot should be restored as much as possible to allow relative ease of future reconstruction. External fixation is often used to supplement the reduction.

Good fluoroscopic imaging is a must for the safe placement of these screws and to make sure the reduction is maintained. These screws can be either solid or cannulated based on the surgeon's preference and comfort. A lag technique works best when the screw is placed perpendicular to a fracture without much comminution. If comminution is present, placement of a fully threaded screw without overdrilling may be preferred just for holding purposes. Placement of a lag screw across comminution may result in compression of the comminuted portion of the fracture and loss of reduction. Similarly, compression that is not perpendicular to the fracture may lead to shearing across the fracture site and loss of reduction. When tightening a screw, one must be aware of the torque that is generated. It is advisable to have a second point of fixation across the fracture to avoid the twisting of the fracture during final tightening. This can be accomplished by placement of a K-wire or a guidewire for a second cannulated screw.

After hardware is placed, meticulous fluoroscopic assessment for intraosseous placement of the hardware is a must. The Canale view must be assessed to confirm there is no penetration of the medial or lateral neck. An ankle mortise view is necessary to make sure there is no intra-articular penetration of medial or lateral talar dome. The lateral view is used to ensure no penetration of the ankle or subtalar joint. AP of the foot evaluates for penetration of the talonavicular joint. Finally, because the talar head is convex, special consideration is needed for talonavicular joint penetration. It is possible to have penetration of that joint that is not picked up on orthogonal radiographs views. The most sensitive view is the one that is perpendicular to the axis of the screw that is being assessed. Multiple live fluoroscopic images are recommended to assess talonavicular articulation.

Postoperatively, the patient is splinted in neutral position for about 2 weeks. Active range of motion can be started thereafter. Weight bearing is initiated 8 to 12 weeks postoperatively depending on radiographic assessment and patient physiology.

Open reduction with internal fixation is used for majority of these injuries. Most of these surgeries are done through dual incisions.

The anteriomedial approach is midway between anterior tibialis and posterior tibialis tendons. It starts distal to talonavicular joint and is extended proximally about 1 to 2 cm proximal to the medial malleolus. Full-thickness flaps are used to dissect down to the joint capsule, and the capsule is incised. The saphenous nerve and vein should be protected. This window can be extended proximally with a medial malleolar osteotomy.[4] Medial malleolar osteotomies can either be chevron shaped or in a single plane at an oblique angle and fixed with two screws after talar fixation is completed.

The anteriolateral approach starts from anterior ankle syndesmosis and proceeds distally toward the base of the fourth metatarsal. Superficially the muscular interval is between extensor digitorium longus and peroneus tertius. Deep to that interval extensor digitorium brevis is identified and retracted plantarly. Superficial peroneal nerve must be identified and protected in this portion of the approach. This can be extended proximally with the lateral malleolar osteotomy.

Of note, if there is a fracture of the distal tibia or fibula present, those fracture can be utilized to improve the exposure of the talus and should typically be fixed after the talar fracture has been addressed.

One should be very careful with soft tissue dissection, particularly plantarly on the medial side in order to preserve vascularity.

Reduction and Internal Fixation Technique

Both approaches described previously are usually needed to judge the reduction. This is because 1 side is usually comminuted, typically medially and dorsally, while the other side is intact. Once both approaches are made, the less comminuted side is used to key in the fracture into reduction. Because of the presence of comminution on the contralateral side of the neck, angulational deformity may persist even with the fracture keyed in on the noncomminuted side of the neck. Careful radiographic assessment is critical on Canale and lateral views. Reduction is provisionally held with K-wires. At times, when there is relatively little comminution, the fracture can be held reduced and compressed with a pointed reduction clam placed through drill holes in the talar neck with the compression vector of the clamp applied perpendicular to the fracture line. However, when segmental comminution is present, it may be necessary to use miniscrews 1.5, 2.0, or 2.4 mm in diameter to fix small comminuted fragments to larger intact fragments in order to be able to judge reduction of the neck.

Occasionally the talar dome is unstable in the ankle mortise. This is common in the presence of a high-grade fracture, Hawkins III, particularly with associated ankle fracture. In that setting, it is difficult to reduce talar head to talar body that is not staying in place. In order to achieve a reduction, it is typically necessary to fix talar dome into its anatomic position in the ankle mortise, usually with multiple 2 mm K-wires.

Internal fixation may be achieved in a similar fashion as described for percutaneous fixation. Portions of navicular may need to be rongeured off in order to allow retrograde placement of screws. When there is no comminution, lag technique should be used to allow fracture compression. When comminution is present, a neutralizing screw without overdrilling needs to be utilized. Lag screws should be placed before neutralizing screws. Alternatively, in the setting of comminution, plates may be placed. On the lateral side there is a large extra-articular concave surface that allows placement of approximately 4-hole 2.0 mm minifragment plate. The plate needs to be contoured to fit the concavity. One must take extra care to ensure that the proximal edge of the plate does not impinge in the ankle joint or that distal end does not to interfere with talonavicular joint, particularly with the distal end of the screws placed into the talar head. On the medial side, a 4-hole minifragment plate can usually be placed just plantar to the cartilage. Similar precautions regarding articular irritation as on the lateral side need to be observed.

Reduction of Extruded Talar Body

A Hawkins III fracture in which the talar dome is extruded posteriormedially is a special situation. These fractures are true emergencies because of the compromise of the soft tissue envelope. Reduction under sedation in the emergency room is nearly impossible. The patient must be taken to the operating room in order to achieve the reduction. These are the author's steps for reducing this injury:

1. The patient is brought to operation room, where anesthesia with muscle paralysis is established. An image intensifier is utilized.
2. The knee is flexed to relax the gastrocnemius.
3. Axial traction is applied to the foot, and gentle anterior pressure is applied to the talus.
4. A centrally threaded pin is placed through the calcaneal tuberosity, and step 3 is repeated while traction is applied through the pin.
5. An anteriolateral approach is performed with direct visualization of the talar dome through the mortise. A Schanz pin is placed into the talar dome to "joystick it," and step 4 is repeated.
6. An anterior medial approach is performed, and step 5 is repeated.
7. A medial malleolar osteotomy is performed, and step 6 is repeated.

The author prefers to do lateral approach first, because the dome is typically extruded posteriormedially and can be better seen from the lateral approach. Some may prefer to perform the medial approach first depending on the soft tissue envelope. Although there have been successful anecdotal experiences of a closed reduction of an extruded talar dome (reduction achieved by step 3 or 4), the author has no personal experience of successful closed reduction of an extruded talus in a patient without concomitant malleolar fracture (this author has not been successful until at least step 5).

The process ends once the talus is reduced. If full exposure is performed, definitive fixation and treatment are performed. If reduction is obtained without open exposure (very unusual), reduction is stabilized with K-wires and external fixator until the definitive e surgery is performed through a dual approach once the swelling decreases. It is important to note that the deltoid attachment to the talar body is the last remnant of blood supply remaining. It cannot be divided in order to achieve reduction (**Figs. 1** and **2**).

LONG-TERM RESULTS

The complications of this injury include AVN, nonunion, malunion, infection, and arthritis of neighboring joints.[5]

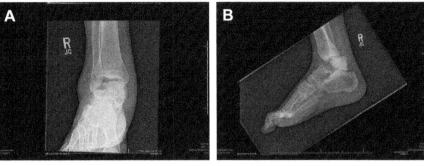

Fig. 1. (A) Anteroposterior and lateral (B) radiograph of a Hawkins 3 talar neck fracture.

AVN is the most common complication. Radiographic presence is not always symptomatic. AVN may consist of a small segment or may result in collapse of the entire talar dome. Incidence of AVN increases as type of fracture increases by Hawkins classification. Some authors recommend use of titanium screws so that MRI of the talus could be obtained to monitor for AVN.[6] Presence of AVN on MRI brings a dilemma

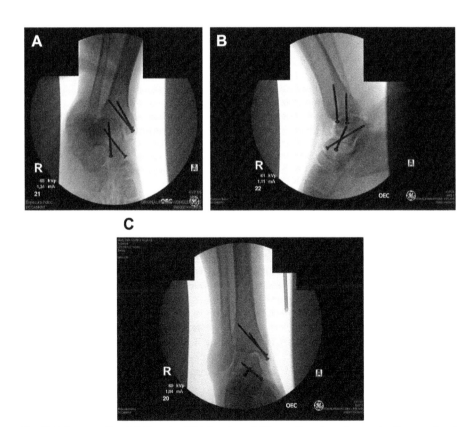

Fig. 2. Intraoperative (A) Canale, (B) lateral, and (C) mortise view demonstrating anatomic reduction of a Hawkins 3 talar neck fracture. Note a medial malleolar osteotomy was required to achieve reduction of the talar body.

of what to do clinically. It is not practical to keep the patient nonweight bearing until the bone revascularizes (could take over 2 years). Some authors suggest patellar tendon-bearing brace to offload the talus. None of these practices have any known clinical benefit and clearly burden the patient. This author uses stainless steel hardware and allows weight bearing after the union is achieved. Once presence of AVN becomes evident, it is treated symptomatically, usually by arthrodesis of the involved joint.[7]

Nonunion is surprisingly uncommon. When it occurs, it may require revision surgery with bone graft. A work-up for infection and a metabolic condition that predisposes for bony nonunion should be preformed. If the patient is a smoker, then a discussion on cessation must be performed.

Work-up for infection consists of clinical assessment of the wound. Infection must be strongly considered in a patient who has had an open injury or a wound that drained for a long period of time postoperatively. Laboratory work consists of sedimentation rate, C-reactive protein, and complete blood cell count (CBC) with differential. If laboratory work is abnormal, or if clinical suspicion is strong, then one should consider white blood cell-tagged bone scan prior to surgery. Intraoperative specimens should be sent to a pathology laboratory to asses for number of white blood cells per high power field and to microbiology for Gram stain and cultures.[8]

Malunion is very common. It occurs in about 30% of cases' this is probably under-reported. Varus malunion is most common, because medial comminution is most common. Not only will this place the hindfoot into varus alignment, but it will also lock subtalar motion, therefore causing the patient to be walking on lateral side of the foot and develop an arthritic subtalar joint.[9] This usually leads to a poor outcome. Treatment is technically challenging, requiring a medial or lateral column lengthening for varus and valgus, malunion respectively.[10] If subtalar arthrosis exists, then an osteotomy is performed along with subtalar fusion.

Infection almost always leads to a poor outcome. It is not uncommon for the soft tissue envelope to be compromised, and a lot of these fractures, particularly Hawkins type III, are open and infection occur frequently.[11] Because the blood supply to the talus is compromised osteomyelitis often develops and is difficult to treat without debridement of dysvascularized bone. In extreme cases, it may require talectomy, placement of antibiotic spacer, and delayed complicated calcaneotibial arthrodesis. In some cases, a below-the-knee amputation may be a preferred reconstructive procedure.

Arthritis of the ankle joint or subtalar joint may develop. It may develop as the result of osteochondral injury, AVN, or malunion. Radiographic evidence of arthritis does not necessarily lead to poor clinical outcome. If the patient is clinically symptomatic, then arthritis is treated in a similar fashion as any arthritis of the involved joint. Options include nonsteroidal anti-inflammatory drugs (NSAIDs), injections, orthoses, and arthrodesis.

TALAR BODY FRACTURES

Body fractures can be in a coronal plane, sagittal plane, or crush injuries.[12]

Sagittal plane fracture can be fixed with screws placed medial to lateral. Screws need to be countersunk deep to the cartilage, or alternatively, headless screws may be used. Exposure is accomplished similar to talar neck. Sometimes it can be done through a single rather than dual approach.

Coronal plane fractures can be treated similar to talar neck if they are relatively distal. Often a malleolar osteotomy is not needed for exposure, and hardware is placed in a similar fashion as for talar neck. When the fracture line is more posterior, then an osteotomy may be necessary.

Crush injuries are often difficult to treat. There are often osteochondral impaction injuries. At times, anatomic reduction may be impossible. Malleolar osteotomy is usually necessary. The surgeon needs to have multiple screws of varied diameter at his or her disposal in order to fix fragments of varied sizes. At the very least joint stability needs to be restored as well as height and length of the talar dome to allow later arthrodesis if becomes necessary. Complications are very similar to talar neck injuries.

Talar Head Fracture

Talar head fractures are hard to see on plane radiographs, and diagnosis is often missed on initial presentation. They may occur with subtalar or midtarsal dislocations. When the fracture appears nondisplaced on plane radiograph, then a CT is recommended to confirm the amount of displacement. A step-off in talonavicular joint is poorly tolerated. Nondisplaced fractures can be treated with 6 weeks of cast immobilization. Displaced small fragments can be excised while larger fragments can be fixed with small screws countersunk beneath the level of the cartilage or with headless screws. The fracture is usually on the medial side, and a single medial approach can be used. In case of significant joint impaction and comminution, bone grafting may be required. If stable reduction is hard to obtain due to impaction or comminution, consider using an external fixator along the medial column, or alternatively, a temporary plate can be used to span the talonavicular joint. The temporary plate or the external fixator is removed at around 6 weeks.

Long-term results are usually good if the fracture was properly diagnosed and treated. Vascularity to the talar head is good, and AVN is not common. Nonunion is rare. Degenerative joint disease may require arthrodesis if conservative care fails. Since stoppage of talonavicular motion will essentially lock subtalar motion, triple arthrodesis is usually preferred to isolated talonavicular fusion (**Figs. 3** and **4**).

LATERAL PROCESS FRACTURES

This is often called a snowboarder's fracture. Patients present with lateral ankle pain, and unfortunately this injury often mistaken for an ankle sprain. It can often be seen on

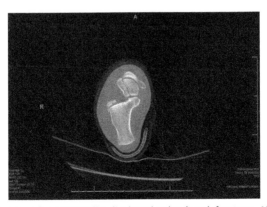

Fig. 3. Axial CT image of a minimally displaced talar head fracture. Note how minimal displacement will likely impinge the talonavicular joint, affecting alignment and motion of the rearfoot.

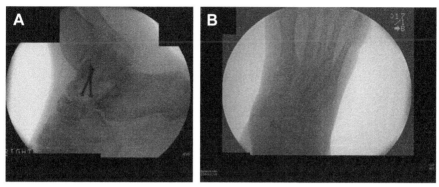

Fig. 4. (*A*) Lateral and (*B*) anteroposterior radiograph of the foot demonstrating open reduction with internal fixation (ORIF) of the same talar head fracture that was performed through a single medial incision.

the mortise view of the ankle. Often a CT is needed to evaluate the size of the fragment and its displacement.

Nondisplaced fragment can be treated nonoperatively with cast immobilization for 6 weeks.

Small displaced fragment can be treated with excision.

Large displaced fragment should be treated with open reduction and internal fixation.

Long-term results of a missed or mistreated injury can result in pain and arthrosis of subtalar joint that may necessitate a subtalar fusion (**Figs. 5** and **6**).

Posterior Process Fractures

The Posterior process has extremely high variability of the anatomy, particularly in size of the medial tubercle and presence absence and size of os trigonum associated with lateral tubercle. May be treated nonoperatively if less than 2 mm of displacement. Otherwise, surgical care is recommended with either excision or open reduction with internal fixation. Excision is utilized when the fragment is small and the patient has either decreased activity level or poor health.

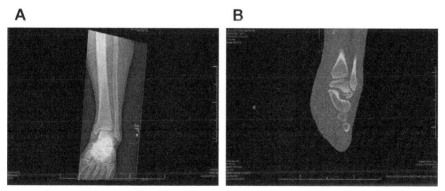

Fig. 5. (*A*) Anteroposterior ankle radiograph and (*B*) CT imaging demonstrating a lateral process fracture of the talus.

A   B

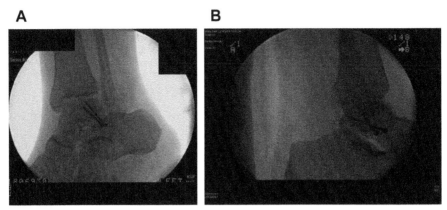

Fig. 6. (A) Intraoperative Canale view and (B) lateral radiograph after osteosynthesis of the same lateral process fracture of the talus.

This portion of the talus has poor vascularity and nonunion is relatively common. Prolonged immobilization beyond 8 weeks may be required.

The posteriolateral tubercle is approached between the tendons of peroneal and flexor hallucis longus. The posteriomedial tubercle is approached around posteriomedial neurovascular bundle. Minifragment screws are used for fixation.

Nonunion is relatively common and may occur in up to 60% of patients treated nonoperatively. Subtalar and ankle joint irritation and arthritis may occur as a result of malreduction, particularly of the larger lateral tubercle.

SUMMARY

Fractures of the talus are relatively rare injuries that usually occur as the result of high energy trauma.

The entire patient needs to be assessed, and more life threatening injuries need to take priority.

The soft tissue envelope around the hindfoot is tenuous and must be protected. At times that may require emergent surgery to reduce and stabilize the bony deformity that is compromising the skin.

Extruded talar body is a special situation and needs to be handled emergently.

Anatomic reduction and rigid fixation is required and performed once swelling subsides, and soft tissue envelope is suitable for surgery.

Complications are common and consist of malunion, arthritis, AVN, and infection.

Once complications occur, the result is usually poor depending on complication. After infection is treated or ruled out the patient may require arthrodesis, osteotomy, and possibly bone grafting to restore the bone stock.

REFERENCES

1. Mulfinger GL, Trueta J. The blood supply of the talus. J Bone Joint Surg Br 1970; 52:160–7.
2. Hawkins LG. Fractures of the neck of the talus. J Bone Joint Surg Am 1970;52: 991–1002.
3. Canale ST, Kelly FB Jr. Fractures of the neck of the talus: long term evaluation of seventy one cases. J Bone Joint Surg Am 1978;60:143–56.

4. Alexander IJ, Watson JT. Step-cut osteotomy of the medial maleolus for exposure of the medial ankle joint space. Foot Ankle 1991;11:242–3.
5. Vallier HA, Nork SE, Barei DP, et al. Talar neck fractures: results and outcomes. J Bone Joint Surg Am 2004;86A:1616–24.
6. Thordarson DB, Trffon MJ, Terk MR. Magnetic resonance imaging to detect avascular necrosis after open reduction and internal fixation of talar neck fractures. Foot Ankle Int 1996;17:742–7.
7. Kitaoka HB, Patzer GL. Arthrodesis for treatment of arthrosis of the ankle and osteonecrosis of the talus. J Bone Joint Surg Am 1998;80:370–9.
8. Migues A, Solari G, Carrasco NM, et al. Repair of talar neck nonunion with indirect corticocancellous graft technique: a case report and review of the literature. Foot Ankle Int 1996;17:690–4.
9. Daniels TR, Smith JW, Roth TI. Varus malalignment of the talar neck: its effect on the position of the foot and subtalar motion. J Bone Joint Surg Am 1996;78:1559–67.
10. Monroe MT, Manoli A II. Osteotomy for malunion of the talar neck fracture: case report. Foot Ankle Int 1999;20:192–5.
11. Sanders R, Pappas J, Mast J, et al. The salvage of open grade IIIB ankle and talas fractures. J Orthop Trauma 1992;6:201–8.
12. Vallier HA, Nork SE, Benirschke SK, et al. Surgical treatment of talar body fractures. J Bone Joint Surg Am 2003;85:1716–24.

Management in High-risk Patients

Patrick Burns, DPM[a],*, Pete Highlander, DPM, MS[a],
Andrew B. Shinabarger, DPM, MS[b]

KEYWORDS

- Polytrauma • Fracture • Diabetes • Charcot • Neuropathy • Osteoporotic • Elderly

KEY POINTS

- Foot and ankle injuries in high-risk populations are associated with poorer outcomes and warrant special attention.
- Foot and ankle injuries in polytraumatized patients are often missed because of more life-threatening injuries and are associated with increased morbidity.
- Fall from height and automobile accidents are a predilection for foot and ankle injuries.
- Staged treatment protocols should be used to optimize the soft tissue envelop and to allow treatment of head and trunk injuries. Fractures in diabetic patients often require more aggressive management.

POLYTRAUMA AND THE FOOT AND ANKLE INJURY

Injuries to the foot and ankle are often missed or underestimated during the initial care of multi-injured patients or patients with polytrauma when life-threatening injuries such as head and trunk injuries or organ dysfunction and respiratory distress syndrome are under control. Many injuries are not realized until later in the patient's hospital stay when weight bearing is attempted. Nonetheless foot and ankle fractures are the source of long-term limitations in polytrauma cases. Multiple studies have analyzed long-term follow-ups and have shown that injures below the knee produce some of the highest rates for unemployment, as well as longer sick leave, more pain, more follow-up appointments, and decreased overall outcome as measured by Short Form 12 instruments.[1–4] Therefore early diagnosis and effective treatment of foot and ankle injuries are imperative. Considering the mechanism of injury may assist in early diagnosis. As noted by Probst and colleagues,[3] polytraumatized patients who

Disclosures: None.
[a] University of Pittsburgh Medical Center Mercy Hospital, Comprehensive Foot and Ankle Center, 1515 Locust Street, #350 Pittsburgh, PA 15219, USA; [b] Legacy Medical Group - Foot and Ankle, 2800 North Vancouver Street, Suite #130, Portland, OR 97229
* University of Pittsburgh Medical Center Mercy Hospital, Comprehensive Foot and Ankle Center, 1515 Locust Street, #350 Pittsburgh, PA 15219, USA.
E-mail address: burnsp@upmc.edu

Clin Podiatr Med Surg 31 (2014) 523–538
http://dx.doi.org/10.1016/j.cpm.2014.06.007
0891-8422/14/$ – see front matter © 2014 Elsevier Inc. All rights reserved.

Evaluation of peripheral neuropathy via meticulous physical examination should be performed for all patients with diabetes. The Michigan Neuropathy Screening Instrument (MNSI) is a validated scoring system that uses assessment of protective sensation, vibratory sensation, and Achilles tendon reflexes to determine the presence or absence of neuropathy.[24,25] In addition, thorough laboratory assessment may also provide additional information necessary for perioperative assessment of any diabetic patient undergoing surgery.[24,26] Shibuya and colleagues[27] analyzed 165 diabetic patients undergoing elective arthrodesis, reconstruction, or ORIF of fractures. There was a statistically significant association for bone healing complication with peripheral neuropathy, surgery duration, and hemoglobin A1c greater than 7%. Tobacco use, documented peripheral arterial disease, body mass index, age, and gender were not statistically significant. History of foot ulceration was statistically significant in bivariate analysis but not in multivariate analysis. In a series of diabetic ankle fractures, Wukich and colleagues[28] showed no statistically significant relationship between complications and age, gender, body mass index, fasting serum glucose, hemoglobin A1c, serum creatinine, and type of fracture.

Blotter and colleagues[29] reported a 43% complication rate for 21 diabetic ankle fractures treated with standard ORIF. Although neuropathy was not quantified using MNSI, 4 of the 21 patients had documented peripheral neuropathy. Two of 4 patients with neuropathy developed serious complications, including septic arthritis, Charcot neuroarthropathy, and osteomyelitis.[29] Kline and colleagues[30] compared complications rates associated with similar surgical methods of pilon fractures for patients with and without diabetes. Overall complication rates were 71% in the diabetic group versus 35% for the nondiabetic group. The diabetic group had an infection rate of 71% compared with a 19% infection rate in nondiabetic patients. Nonunion or delayed union was also higher in the diabetic group compared with the nondiabetic group: 43% versus 16%, respectively. Neuropathy was not measured for any of the patients.[30] Jones and colleagues[31] retrospectively reviewed 42 diabetic ankle fractures. Twenty-one of the patients had documented complicated diabetes and the remaining 21 had uncomplicated diabetes. Both groups underwent similar surgical management. The complicated diabetic population had a 47% complication rate compared with 14% complication rate in those patients with uncomplicated diabetes. The investigators found an association between the development of Charcot neuroarthropathy and patients with peripheral neuropathy and nephropathy. They also noted a trend toward postoperative infection and nephropathy.[31]

Neuropathic ankle fractures have been the subject of much research in the last decade. Multiple studies have suggested the need for additional fixation and more detailed postoperative protocols. Marks[32] proposed that patients with peripheral neuropathy should have their postoperative immobilization period increased 2-fold to 3-fold, which is a protocol shared by other investigators.[28,33] Wukich and colleagues[28] noted that some diabetic patients may be unable to comply with prolonged weight-bearing status given reduced cardiovascular reserve, neuropathy, balance issues, obesity, and upper extremity weakness. According to the investigators, these patients may benefit from circular ring external fixation in addition to ORIF constructs to protect osseous reduction.[28] Pinzur[34] noted this strategy was successful for Charcot reconstructions.

Pinzur[35] also reported on 5 diabetic patients with loss of protective sensation who sustained symptomatic malunited stress fracture of the distal tibia. Two of the patients failed standard ORIF of ankle fractures and 3 failed closed management. All 5 patients were successfully treated with transarticular stabilization with antegrade or retrograde intramedullary nailing.

Wukich and colleagues[28] analyzed results from 105 diabetic ankle fractures. Complicated diabetic patients had a 3.8-times higher risk of overall complications, 3.4-times higher noninfectious complications (malunion, nonunion, or Charcot neuroarthropathy), and 5-times higher infectious complications compared with their uncomplicated counterparts. When the researchers compared fixation constructs, the ORIF-plus group, defined by standard ORIF construct with the addition of tetracortical syndesmotic screw and/or transarticular pin fixation (**Fig. 1**), had a statistically significant lower complication rate compared with standard ORIF alone: 5.7% versus 20% respectively. The ORIF and external fixation construct group had a 54.3% complication rate, of which most were pin tract infections, and open fractures were included within this group.[28]

Patients with diabetes may be prone to calcaneal fractures resulting from systemic factors as well as spontaneous or insufficiency fractures.[36–38] Insufficiency fractures, which resemble avulsion fractures, have been treated with excision of the fracture fragment and reattachment of the Achilles tendon with double-row anchor fixation with good clinical outcomes (**Fig. 2**).[36] Primary subtalar joint arthrodesis may be a treatment of choice for high-grade, comminuted calcaneal fractures especially in the setting of diabetes, peripheral neuropathy, and obesity.[38,39] Primary arthrodesis should be considered in cases of high-grade fractures, extensive comminution, and joint involvement, as well as in the setting of peripheral neuropathy when development of Charcot neuroarthropathy is possible (**Fig. 3**). Given the plethora of literature in animal and human models suggesting increased bone healing complications in diabetic and neuropathic fractures,[27,29,31,33,36,40–44] alternative fixation constructs for all types of diabetic fractures should be considered.

MANAGEMENT OF FOOT AND ANKLE FRACTURES IN THE GERIATRIC POPULATION

Estimates state that by the year 2035 almost 20% of the US population will be 65 years of age and older.[45] This age group currently continues to have improved health, better mobility, and a more active lifestyle compared with the same age group in the past. The increased activity level and continued high physical demand has the potential to lead to an increase in high-energy trauma. Patients more than 65 years of age account for 23% of all trauma admissions, and trauma is the fifth largest cause of death in this population.[46,47] However, inadequate data exist regarding high-energy skeletal trauma care in the elderly, with even less literature dedicated to the management of the distal lower extremity.[48] Several major implications need to be taken into account when dealing with high-energy injuries to the foot and ankle in the elderly population.

The outcome of trauma in the elderly patient often begins with the initial triage. The importance of transfer to a designated trauma center has been well documented in this patient population. Alas, several studies have shown that elderly trauma victims are often undertriaged, which has prompted many researchers to suggest that the elderly should only be referred to dedicated trauma centers.[48–52] After initial triage, aggressive resuscitation should be performed if necessary because hypotension and hypoperfusion are underestimated in the elderly population.[48] Once patients are stabilized, the next step is to survey their overall medical state, because numerous medical comorbidities can complicate patient management and overall recovery. Clinicians should remember that more than 50% of geriatric patients with trauma have hypertension and more than 30% have heart disease.[46,53] Other common conditions that can complicate evaluation and management are diabetes mellitus, history of cerebrovascular accident, cancer, hepatic disease, dementia, arrhythmias, chronic obstructive pulmonary disease, and others. Because of compounding medical

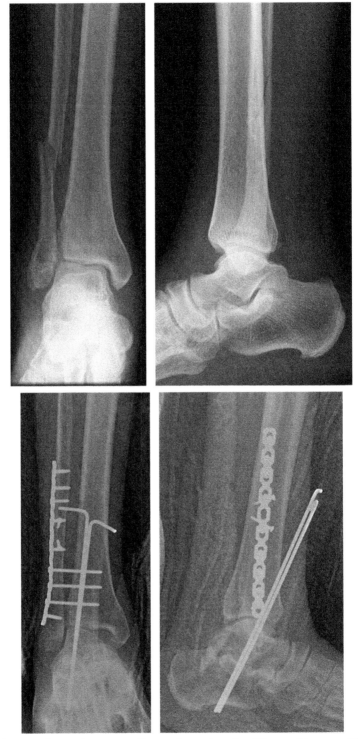

Fig. 1. Preoperative and postoperative radiographs of a 79-year-old man with insulin-dependent diabetes, peripheral neuropathy (MNSI, 6/10), nephropathy on dialysis who sustained an ankle fracture after a slip and fall on ice. The ORIF-plus construct is depicted in the immediate postoperative films with transarticular pins and multiple syndesmotic screw fixation.

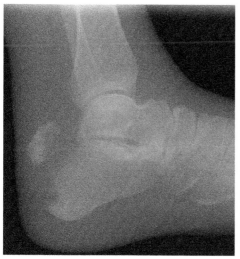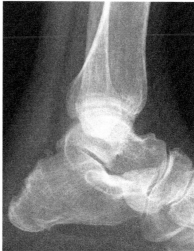

Fig. 2. Preoperative and postoperative radiographs of a 49-year-old woman with insulin-dependent diabetes and peripheral neuropathy (MNSI, 6/10) felt a pop over her heel while walking. Calcaneal avulsion/insufficiency fracture, also known as calcaneal Charcot neuro-arthropathy. The patient was successfully treated with detachment of the Achilles tendon, excision of the fracture fragment, and reattachment of the Achilles tendon with a double-row anchor fixation construct.

factors, comorbidities, and polypharmacy, having a geriatrician involved in the management of the patient has been shown to decrease length of stay, readmission rates, complication rates, and patient mortality.[48,54,55]

Ground-level falls followed by motor vehicle accident are the most common causes of injury in the geriatric population.[56] However, with the increased activity of geriatrics, falls from greater heights, such as from ladders or trees, may become more prevalent. The injury pattern of older individuals is often disproportionate to the mechanism of injury because of altered bone metabolism associated with osteopenia and osteoporosis.[56] Low-energy mechanisms causing high-grade fractures in this patient population often require surgical intervention (**Fig. 4**), with the cited rates being as high as 92%.[57] Ankle fractures rank as the third most common fracture in geriatrics, following hip and wrist fractures.[58] Herscovici and Scaduto[57] analyzed 243 geriatric foot and ankle fractures and discovered that ankle fractures were the most common encountered. These were followed in decreasing occurrence by calcaneal fractures, pilon fractures, talus fractures, metatarsal fractures, midfoot fractures, Lisfranc injuries, and pure foot dislocations.

Conventional treatment modalities have limited success in the geriatric population because of soft tissue integrity, poor bone quality, intrinsic instability, and compliance difficulties with weight-bearing restrictions.[59] Contraindications for foot and ankle surgery in the elderly include bed-bound or chair-bound patients, severe peripheral vascular disease, medical problems that preclude patients from surgery, and cognitive issues that cause noncompliance issues resulting in high failure rates. However, withholding surgical intervention from an elderly patient who presents with a high-energy injury can also result in significant problems, because nonoperative management frequently leads to debilitating outcomes.[57] Thus for patients not mentioned in one of the groups mentioned earlier, operative management for high-grade injuries of the foot and ankle should be considered.

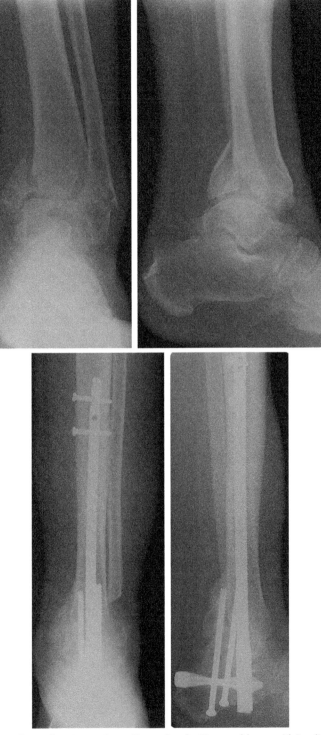

Fig. 3. Preoperative and postoperative radiographs of a 62-year-old man with insulin-dependent diabetes, peripheral neuropathy (MNSI, 7/10), nephropathy on hemodialysis, and history of a heart transplant who had an ankle that was treated nonoperatively by an outside physician. The patient developed Charcot neuroarthropathy associated with deformity. The patient was treated successfully with a single-staged tibiotalocalcaneal arthrodesis with intramedullary fixation.

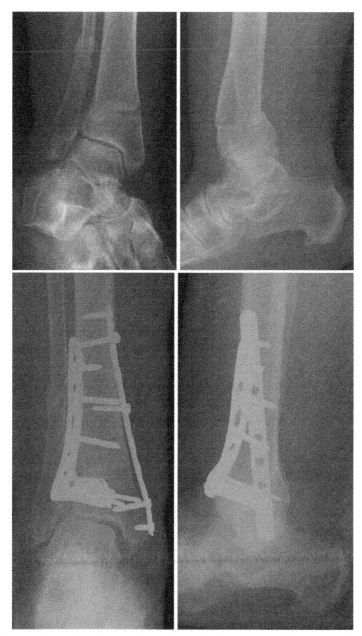

Fig. 4. Preoperative and postoperative radiographs of a 74-year-old woman with osteopenia and hypertension who developed a distal tibial and fibular stress fracture. With no apparent injury, the patient noticed increasing deformity, pain, and difficulty ambulating.

Soft tissue management is of paramount importance for any high-grade fracture and may be even more critical in elderly patients, who often have thin atrophic skin, questionable soft tissue envelope, and impaired microcirculation. Prompt anatomic reduction and well-padded splint application are crucial to decrease skin tension in

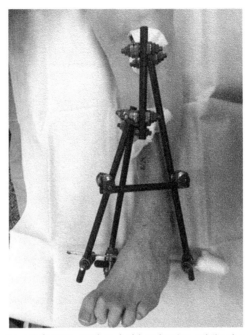

Fig. 5. Pin to bar external fixator used to hold reduction while the soft tissue envelope improves.

a timely fashion. For exceptionally unstable fracture or when reduction maintenance is not amendable to splint immobilization, operative fixation is indicated. Temporizing these fractures with external fixation provides excellent stability and allows for close soft tissue monitoring (**Fig. 5**). In these cases, definitive internal fixation is placed when the zone of soft tissue injury subsides, which is often 7 to 21 days after initial injury. Geriatric fractures are often amendable to less invasive stabilizations system plating or minimally invasive plate osteosynthesis. These techniques preserve soft tissue and blood supply to the area by using a limited surgical exposure (**Fig. 6**). Another adjunct commonly used in this patient population is incisional negative pressure

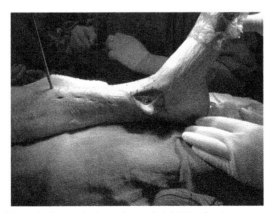

Fig. 6. Limited-incision plating technique for a distal tibia fracture.

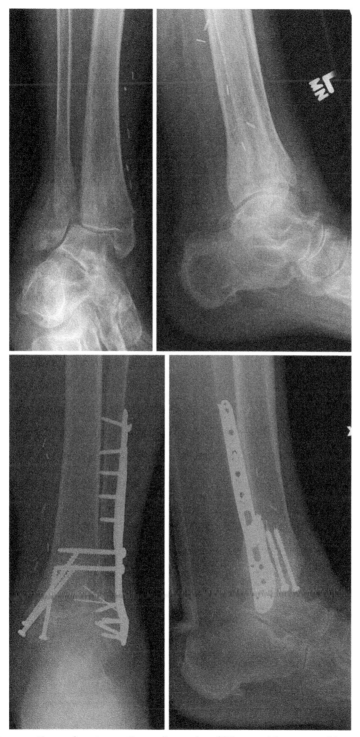

Fig. 7. Preoperative and postoperative radiographs of 88-year-old woman with osteopenia, hypothyroid, hypertension, and coronary artery disease who sustained a bimalleolar ankle fracture from a ground-level fall. A relative stability fibular construct was used with locking plate and syndesmotic screws.

wound therapy, which has been shown to decrease incisional complications and aid in reduction of hematoma and seroma formation.[60,61]

Another difficulty of which the surgeon must be aware in this patient population is osteoporosis or osteopenic bone, which is the most common disease of the bone. Osteoporosis is characterized by low bone mass, deterioration of bone tissue, increased fragility, and a higher risk of fracture leading to approximately 2.1 million osteoporotic fractures yearly in the United States.[59,62] The decrease in bone quality not only leads to fractures; it may lead to complications with fixation. The concept of locked plating is often recommended in this population because it provides several advantages compared with traditional plating systems (**Fig. 7**). The suggested benefits of locking plate technology include the improved biology of fracture healing and improved biomechanics of fracture fixation.[63] Reduced disruption of the soft tissue envelope and periosteal vascular supply are achieved via minimally invasive plating techniques and limited-contact plate designs, as well as by the ability to achieve stable constructs without relying on friction at the plate-bone interface. From a mechanical standpoint, locking plates or relative stability constructs behave differently compared with conventional nonlocking or absolute stability constructs. Without the motion at each individual screw-plate junction that occurs in nonlocked constructs, locking constructs can be modeled as single-beam constructs or a fixed-angle device, which are significantly more stable.[63–67] In addition, external fixation for osteoporotic fractures should be considered because it may allow for earlier patient mobility, thereby limiting deconditioning and associated complications.

Management of high-grade injuries to the foot and ankle in the geriatric patient can be difficult. By adhering to proper soft tissue handling while providing adequate fixation and managing medical comorbidities many complications may be avoided. Surgical reconstruction for high-grade fractures in geriatric patients should be considered a viable option in order to restore the anatomy, regain early function, and avoid complications seen with the nonoperative care of these injuries. Results from several studies show that surgery for injuries of the foot and ankle in the elderly have similar outcomes and complications to those seen in younger patients.[57,68–72]

SUMMARY

Foot and ankle injuries in high-risk populations are associated with poorer outcomes and warrant special attention in high-risk populations. Foot and ankle injuries in polytraumatized patients are often missed because of more life-threatening injuries and are associated with increased morbidity. Fall from height and automobile accidents are predilections for foot and ankle injuries. Staged treatment protocols should be used to optimize the soft tissue envelop and to allow for treatment of head and trunk injuries. Fractures in diabetic patients often require more aggressive management. Documentation of neuropathy by the MNSI should be used because it places patients in a heightened risk category. Development of a Charcot joint and deformity often occurs even when standard open reduction and fixation techniques are used. To prevent this, research has suggested more rigid fixation constructs and primary arthrodesis for neuropathic fractures. Increased mobility and longevity of the elderly places these patients at increased risk for fracture. Ground-level falls followed by automobile accidents are the most common causes for geriatric fractures. Bone and soft tissue are of inferior quality. More rigid fixation constructs should be used for osteoporotic fractures. Soft tissue envelopes are often atrophic and have poor microcirculation, therefore careful, atraumatic soft tissue handling is of extreme importance. In addition, attention to medical comorbidities and polypharmacy promotes the safety of the geriatric patient during the perioperative period.

REFERENCES

1. Butcher JL, MacKenzie EJ, Cushing B, et al. Long-term outcomes after lower extremity trauma. J Trauma 1996;41:4–9.
2. Mackenzie EJ, Bosse MJ, Castillo RC, et al. Functional outcomes following trauma-related lower-extremity amputation. J Bone Joint Surg Am 2004;86: 1636–45.
3. Probst C, Pape HC, Hildebrand F, et al. 30 years of polytrauma care: an analysis of the change in strategies and results of 4,849 cases treated at a single institution. Injury 2009;40:77–83.
4. Zelle BA, Brown SR, Panzica M, et al. The impact of injuries below the knee joint on the long-term functional outcome following polytrauma. Injury 2005;36:169–77.
5. Probst C, Richter M, Lefering R, et al. Incidence and significance of injuries to the foot and ankle in polytrauma patients – an analysis of the trauma registry of DGU. Injury 2010;41:210–5.
6. Kinzl L, Gebhard F, Liener UC, et al. Trauma surgery 2020. Past developments – future demand and perspectives. III. Ideas on future care. Unfallchirurg 1999; 102:371–4.
7. Richter M, Thermann H, Wippermann B, et al. Foot fractures in restrained front seat car occupants: a long-term study over twenty-three years. J Orthop Trauma 2001;15:287–93.
8. Gardner MJ, Demetrakopoulous D, Briggs SM, et al. The ability of the Lauge-Hansen classification to predict ligament injury and mechanism in ankle fractures: an MRI study. J Orthop Trauma 2006;20:267–72.
9. Attinger CE, Evans KK, Bulan E, et al. Angiosomes of the foot and ankle and clinical implications for limb salvage: reconstruction, incisions, and revascularization. Plast Reconstr Surg 2006;117:261S–93S.
10. Pape HC, Giannoudis P, Krettek C. The timing of fracture treatment in polytrauma patients: relevance of damage control orthopedic surgery. Am J Surg 2002;183:622–9.
11. Aktuglu K, Aydogan U. The functional outcome of displace intra-articular calcaneal fractures: a comparison between isolate cases and polytrauma patients. Foot Ankle Int 2002;23:314–8.
12. Harris AM, Patterson BM, Sontich JK, et al. Results and outcomes after operative treatment of high-energy tibial plafond fractures. Foot Ankle Int 2006;27:256–65.
13. Thornton SJ, Cheleuitte D, Ptaszek AJ, et al. Treatment of open intra-articular calcaneal fractures: evaluation of treatment protocol based on wound location and size. Foot Ankle Int 2006;27:317–23.
14. Sirkin M, Sanders R, DiPasquale T, et al. A staged protocol for soft tissue management in the treatment of complex pilon fractures. J Orthop Trauma 1999;18: S32–8.
15. Acott AA, Theus SA, Kim LT. Long-term glucose control and risk of perioperative complications. Am J Surg 2009;198:596–9.
16. Dronge AS, Perkal MF, Kancir S, et al. Long-term glycemic control and postoperative infectious complications. Arch Surg 2006;141:375–80.
17. Golden SH, Peart-Vigilance C, Kao WH, et al. Perioperative glycemic control and the risk of infectious complications in a cohort of adults with diabetes. Diabetes Care 1999;22:1408–14.

18. Myers TG, Lowery NJ, Frykberg RG, et al. Ankle and hindfoot fusions: comparison of outcomes in patient with and without diabetes. Foot Ankle Int 2012; 33(20):20–8.
19. Perlman MH, Thordarson DB. Ankle fusion in a high risk population: an assessment of nonunion risk factors. Foot Ankle Int 1999;20:491–6.
20. Wukich DK, Belczyk RJ, Burns PR, et al. Complications encountered with circular ring fixation in persons with diabetes mellitus. Foot Ankle Int 2008;29: 994–1000.
21. Wukich DK, Shen JY, Ramirez CP, et al. Retrograde ankle arthrodesis using and intramedullary nail: a comparison of patients with and without diabetes. J Foot Ankle Surg 2011;50:299–306.
22. Younger AS, Awwad MA, Kalla TP, et al. Risk factors for failure of transmetatarsal amputation in diabetic patients: a cohort study. Foot Ankle Int 2009;30: 1177–82.
23. Bax G, Fagherazzi C, Piarulli F, et al. Reproducibility of Michigan Neuropathy Screening Instrument (MNSI). A comparison with tests using the vibratory and thermal perception thresholds. Diabetes Care 1996;19:904–5.
24. Highlander P, Shinabarger AB. Perioperative laboratory assessment of diabetic foot infections undergoing amputation: a systematic review. Foot Ankle Spec 2013;6:465–70.
25. Wukich DK, Hobizal KB, Raspovic KM, et al. SIRS is valid in discriminating between severe and moderate diabetic foot infections. Diabetes Care 2013;36: 3706–11.
26. Moghtaderi A, Bakhshipour A, Rashidi H. Validation of Michigan neuropathy screening instrument for diabetic peripheral neuropathy. Clin Neurol Neurosurg 2006;108:477–81.
27. Shibuya N, Humphers JM, Fluhman BL, et al. Factors associated with nonunion, delayed union and malunion in foot and ankle surgery in diabetic patients. J Foot Ankle Surg 2013;52:207–11.
28. Wukich DK, Joseph A, Ryan M, et al. Outcomes of ankle fractures in patients with uncomplicated versus complicated diabetes. Foot Ankle Int 2011;32: 120–30.
29. Blotter RH, Connolly E, Wasan A, et al. Acute complications in the operative treatment of isolated ankle fractures in patients with diabetes mellitus. Foot Ankle Int 1999;20:687–94.
30. Kline AJ, Gruen GS, Pape HC, et al. Early complications following the operative treatment of pilon fractures with and without diabetes. Foot Ankle Int 2009;30: 1042–7.
31. Jones KB, Maiers-Yelden KA, Marsh JL, et al. Ankle fractures in patients with diabetes mellitus. J Bone Joint Surg Br 2005;87:489–95.
32. Marks RM. Complications of foot and ankle surgery in patients with diabetes. Clin Orthop Rel Res 2001;391:153–61.
33. Costigan W, Thordarson DB, Debnath UK. Operative management of ankle fractures in patients with diabetes mellitus. Foot Ankle Int 2007;28:32–7.
34. Pinzur MS. Neutral ring fixation for high-risk nonplantigrade Charcot midfoot deformity. Foot Ankle Int 2007;28:961–6.
35. Pinzur MS. Transarticular stabilization for malunited fracture of the distal tibia in diabetics with loss of protective sensation. Foot Ankle Int 2001;22:706–10.
36. Greenhagen RM, Highlander PD, Burns PR. Double row anchor fixation: a novel technique for a diabetic calanceal insufficiency avulsion fracture. J Foot Ankle Surg 2012;51:123–7.

37. Kathol MH, El-Khoury GY, Moore TE, et al. Calcaneal insufficiency avulsion fractures in patients with diabetes mellitus. Radiology 1991;180:725–9.
38. Facaros Z, Ramanujam CL, Zgonis T. Primary subtalar joint arthrodesis with internal and external fixation for the repair of a diabetic comminuted calcaneal fracture. Clin Podiatr Med Surg 2011;28:203–9.
39. Stapleton JJ, Kolodenker G, Zgonis T. Internal and external fixation approaches to the surgical management of calcaneal fractures. Clin Podiatr Med Surg 2010; 27:381–92.
40. Levitt BA, Stapleton JJ, Zgonis T. Diabetic Lisfranc fracture-dislocations and Charcot neuroarthropathy. Clin Podiatr Med Surg 2013;30:257–63.
41. Alblowi J, Kayal RA, Siqueria M, et al. High levels of tumor necrosis factor-alpha contribute to accelerated loss of cartilage in diabetic fracture healing. Am J Pathol 2009;175:1574–85.
42. Follak N, Kloting I, Merk H. Influence of diabetic metabolic state on fracture healing in spontaneously diabetic rats. Diabetes Metab Res Rev 2005;21: 288–96.
43. Gandhi A, Liporace F, Azad V, et al. Diabetic fracture healing. Foot Ankle Clin 2006;11:805–24.
44. Bibbo C, Lin SS, Beam HA, et al. Complications of ankle fractures in diabetic patients. Orthop Clin North Am 2001;32:113–33.
45. United States Census Bureau. Projections of the population by selected age groups and sex for the United States: 2010 to 2050, 2011. Available at: http://www.census.gov/population/projections/data/national/2012.html.
46. Bonne S, Schuerer DJ. Trauma in the older adult, epidemiology and evolving geriatric trauma principles. Clin Geriatr Med 2013;29:137–50.
47. Keller JM, Sciadini MF, Sinclair E, et al. Geriatric trauma: demographics, injuries and mortality. J Orthop Trauma 2012;26:161–5.
48. Switzer JA, Gammon SR. High-energy skeletal trauma in the elderly. J Bone Joint Surg Am 2012;94:2195–204.
49. Jacobs DG, Plaisier BR, Barie PS, et al. Practice management guidelines for geriatric trauma: the EAST practice management guidelines work group. J Trauma 2003;54:391–416.
50. Jacos DG. Special considerations in geriatric injury. Curr Opin Crit Care 2003; 9(6):535–9.
51. Moore L, Turgeon AF, Sirois MJ, et al. Trauma centre outcome performance: a comparison of young adults and geriatric patients in an inclusive trauma system. Injury 2012;43:1580–5.
52. Mann NC, Cahn RM, Mullins RJ, et al. Survival among injured geriatric patients during construction of a statewide trauma system. J Trauma 2001;50:1111–6.
53. Thompson HJ, McCormick WC, Kagan SH. Traumatic brain injury in older adults: epidemiology, outcomes, and future implications. J Am Geriatr Soc 2006;54:1590–5.
54. Friedman SM, Mendelson DA, Bingham KW, et al. Impact of a co-managed geriatric fracture center on short-term hip fracture outcomes. Arch Intern Med 2009; 169(18):1712–7.
55. Kates SL, Mendelson DA, Friedman SM. The value of an organized fracture program for the elderly: early results. J Orthop Trauma 2011;25:233–7.
56. Sterling DA, O'Connor JA, Bonadies J. Geriatric falls: injury severity is high and disproportionate to mechanism. J Trauma 2001;50:116–9.
57. Herscovici DJ, Scaduto JM. Management of high-energy foot and ankle injuries in the geriatric population. Geriatr Orthop Surg Rehabil 2012;3:33–44.

exists. The degree of fracture displacement and/or comminution along with the extent of soft tissue injury has to be evaluated. A high index of suspicion is paramount for associated body injuries, including fractures of the lumbar spine and concomitant lower extremity fractures.

Evaluation of certain patient characteristics may affect the surgical approach or decision making toward a nonoperative treatment. Patients with uncontrolled diabetes mellitus, severe peripheral arterial disease in the presence of dense peripheral neuropathy, and existence of multiple medical comorbidities may require particular attention to the overall management of calcaneal fractures. In certain case scenarios, limited open reduction and internal fixation techniques, closed reduction, percutaneous pinning, external fixation, and/or delayed primary subtalar joint arthrodesis may be performed among this complex patient population.[1,2] Medical optimization of severely uncontrolled diabetic patients with multiple comorbidities and vascular surgery consultation in the presence of critical limb ischemia is paramount in cases when operative treatment might be necessary.

Plain radiographic evaluation of calcaneal fractures includes a lateral view of the hindfoot and ankle, anteroposterior view of the foot, axial view of the calcaneus, and anteroposterior and mortise views of the ankle. The lateral view of the hindfoot and ankle typically reveals most of the displaced intra-articular calcaneal fractures. The lateral view will reveal joint-depressed and tongue-type fractures that involve the posterior facet of the subtalar joint. The anteroposterior view of the foot will detect calcaneal fractures that extend into the calcaneocuboid joint. The axial view of the calcaneus reveals the associated widening of the calcaneus, medial wall, and displacement of the tuberosity (typically varus angulation and shortening), with limited evaluation of fractures involving the sustentaculum tali. The anteroposterior view of the ankle will reveal avulsion rim fractures of the fibula, suggesting possible peroneal tendon subluxation, whereas the mortise view of the ankle will reveal the involvement of the posterior facet of the subtalar joint. Once an intra-articular calcaneal fracture is detected on plain radiographs, a computed tomography (CT) scan is required to adequately evaluate the fracture pattern. The coronal views are performed perpendicular to the posterior articular surface of the subtalar joint. Understanding the anatomic variants of calcaneal fractures is paramount to achieving proper anatomic fracture reduction and to aid in the diagnosis and prognosis of the patients' outcomes.

The timing of surgery is determined by the evaluation of the soft tissue envelope and the anticipated surgical approach to achieve fracture reduction. When an extensile lateral approach is to be performed, surgical reconstruction may have to be delayed until the associated edema has subsided. The soft tissue envelope is evaluated for the presence of skin lines, a positive pinch test (the ability to pinch the skin over the proposed incision), and presence of fracture blisters if present. Edema control should be obtained through strict elevation of the lower extremity at rest and layered compression dressings. If a minimal incisional approach is to be performed, surgical reconstruction may be considered sooner because a delay in treatment with a minimal incisional approach may increase the risk for malreduction.

OPEN CALCANEAL FRACTURES

Open calcaneal fractures can present with simple to complex wounds, neurovascular injury, and/or osseous defects. Open fracture treatment protocols may include and are not limited to intravenous antibiosis, tetanus prophylaxis, irrigation and thorough wound debridement, fracture stabilization, delayed wound closure, and delayed osseous reconstruction. A standardized approach to open calcaneal fractures is paramount to minimize postoperative complications.

Most often, open calcaneal fractures are associated with a simple medial wound that can be closed following serial debridements. Simple wounds are usually linear traumatic small lacerations and without any evidence of nerve or arterial injury. Complex wounds are usually very large in size and may involve the plantar surface of the foot, are associated with nerve and/or arterial injury that may require free tissue transfer, and may present with degloving injuries of the heel pad. The wounds associated with open calcaneal fractures are usually covered with standard moist to dry dressings versus an application of negative-pressure wound therapy after the initial debridement and irrigation. Wound closure is usually delayed after a series of irrigation and debridement procedures if the wound is simple, clean, and can be closed without significant tension (**Fig. 1**). Complex wounds with soft tissue loss may require delayed soft tissue coverage using split-thickness skin grafts and/or free flap coverage.

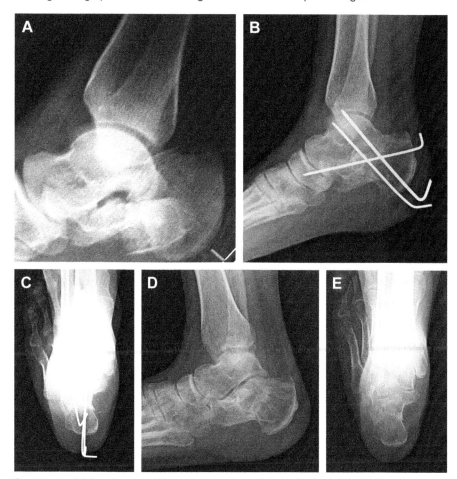

Fig. 1. Lateral (*A*) radiograph of an open displaced intra-articular joint-depressed calcaneal fracture. Reduction was performed through the medial open fracture wound 48 hours after the initial surgical debridement. Postoperative lateral (*B*) and calcaneal axial (*C*) radiographs demonstrating reduction with percutaneous transarticular pinning. Final lateral (*D*) and calcaneal axial (*E*) radiographs demonstrating the alignment and osseous union.

Fracture stabilization for an open calcaneal fracture can be performed with external fixation and/or Steinmann pins. Delayed open reduction and internal fixation can be performed in weeks from the initial injury and if the soft tissue envelope permits with similar outcomes to closed calcaneal fractures. If external fixation is applied, careful attention has to be made to the placement of pins into the calcaneus. An external fixator can be applied with tibio-metatarsal transfixation avoiding the calcaneus, but this form of fixation often only limits the Achilles contracture on the heel. Meticulous placement of calcaneal transfixation must consider the fracture pattern and definitive fracture management.

At times, fracture reduction using a medial approach through the open medial wound, if present, can be performed. Internal fixation can be placed at the time of wound closure, and/or definitive fixation can be achieved by reducing the medial wall and posterior facet of the subtalar joint. This technique allows for adequate fracture reduction and stability while minimizing further soft tissue injury. Limitations with this technique include not addressing the lateral wall widening and depressed and/or displaced superolateral fracture fragments involving the posterior facet of the subtalar joint. In certain cases, a second small lateral sinus tarsi incision can be used to facilitate the reduction of the superolateral fracture fragment of the posterior facet and to facilitate the intra-articular joint reduction.

Prolonged delay of treatment can lead to posttraumatic calcaneal reconstruction that is focused on realignment calcaneal osteotomies, decompression ostectomy of the lateral wall and subtalar joint in situ, or distraction arthrodesis combined with adjunctive soft tissue procedures to address concomitant peroneal tendon pathology.

MINIMAL INCISION VERSUS EXTENSILE LATERAL APPROACH

Minimal incision techniques are used when urgent reduction and fracture stabilization is required because of soft tissue compromise from severely displaced fracture fragments or when associated with rare calcaneal dislocations. This technique can be performed with closed, percutaneous, and limited incision reduction and pinning (**Fig. 2**). In addition, fracture reduction can be supplemented with external fixation and before the definitive open treatment is performed. Definitive fixation with percutaneous screws can be performed if anatomic reduction is achieved and usually in the presence of tongue-type calcaneal fractures. The minimal incisional approach involves

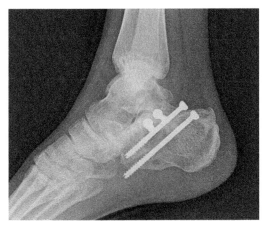

Fig. 2. Lateral postoperative radiograph demonstrating reduction of a calcaneal fracture with a minimal incision approach and placement of cannulated screws.

the utilization of small incisions for percutaneous placement of fixation, a sinus tarsi incision, and/or a medial incision.[3]

A minimal incisional approach is suitable for certain intra-articular calcaneal fracture patterns. Tongue-type fractures that involve only 2 fracture fragments of the posterior facet may be reduced with a minimal incisional approach. In addition, minimally displaced intra-articular fractures of the posterior facet can be reduced with a minimal incisional approach and if the soft tissue envelope allows for timely intervention. Tongue-type fractures should be confirmed on CT images to determine that the displaced intra-articular fracture fragment is attached to the posterior superior calcaneal tuberosity. CT images also allow the surgeon the ability to evaluate the displacement of the medial wall and alignment across the primary fracture line among joint-depressed fractures to determine if an indirect reduction can be achieved.

The extensile lateral approach still remains the gold standard for the operative management of intra-articular calcaneal fractures (**Fig. 3**). The advantages to an extensile lateral approach include direct anatomic reduction of the posterior facet and calcaneal body. In addition, the peroneal tendons can be inspected for subluxation and repaired

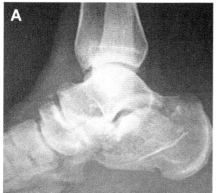
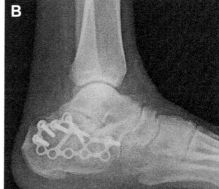
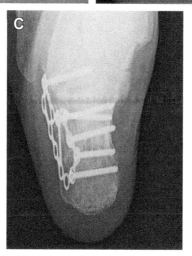

Fig. 3. Lateral (A) radiograph demonstrating an intra-articular joint-depressed calcaneal fracture. Long-term lateral (B) and (C) calcaneal axial radiographs demonstrating anatomic reduction achieved with an extensile lateral approach.

if required. This approach is usually indicated in the 3-part fractures of the posterior facet of the subtalar joint, joint-depressed fractures, significant shortening and varus position of the calcaneal tuberosity, and displacement of the medial wall and is delayed in treatment fractures that require a larger surgical incision to achieve proper anatomic alignment.

POSTOPERATIVE COMPLICATIONS

Calcaneal fractures can be associated with various complications, including wound dehiscence and infection. Superficial wound dehiscence without drainage or exposed hardware is typically managed with frequent local wound care treatments and oral antibiotics. The presence of a hematoma should be managed with early incision and drainage to avoid soft tissue loss and/or deep infection. Purulent drainage should be addressed with early irrigation and debridement along with intraoperative cultures to guide antibiotic treatment. Retained hardware may be maintained if the hardware is stable without subsidence and the infection is addressed acutely. Initial wound management typically involves the utilization of negative-pressure wound therapy. Delayed primary closure can be performed if the surgical wound can be reapproximated with minimal tension. For larger soft tissue defects with exposed hardware, early flap coverage should be performed once the infection has been addressed and after meticulous debridement of all nonviable tissues. Wounds with exposed hardware and deep structures mandate early surgical debridement and soft tissue coverage to avoid limb loss.

The surgical management of a calcaneal malunion and/or posttraumatic subtalar joint arthritis is managed with realignment calcaneal osteotomies and subtalar versus triple arthrodesis, respectively. The goal of a calcaneal osteotomy is to realign the weight-bearing axis of the calcaneus to the lower leg. Most commonly, a calcaneal varus malunion will require a closing wedge or lateral displacement calcaneal osteotomy to reestablish this alignment. A neglected lateral calcaneal wall blowout will result in a widened heel along with possible peroneal tendon entrapment or subluxation. A lateral wall calcaneal ostectomy can adequately address the malunited lateral wall and decompress the peroneal tendons. Peroneal tendon subluxation, if present, can be addressed with reconstruction of the superior peroneal retinaculum with a fibular groove deepening when performed independently. However, when combined with calcaneal osteotomies, ostectomies, and/or subtalar joint arthrodesis, a lateral ankle reconstruction by using a split portion of the peroneal brevis or longus is required to address the peroneal tendon subluxation.

Subtalar joint arthrodesis can be performed in situ to address symptomatic posttraumatic arthritis without malalignment. Joint depression involves a subtalar joint bone block distraction arthrodesis. A subtalar joint arthrodesis can be performed in conjunction with a calcaneal osteotomy, ostectomy, and adjunctive soft tissue procedures.[4]

DISCUSSION

Displaced intra-articular calcaneal fractures are commonly associated with some form of functional limitations and discomfort postoperatively. The severity of the initial injury has been historically determined by the degree of impaction of the posterior facet of the subtalar joint and quantified by measuring the Bohler angle (plain radiographs) and Sanders classification through CT imaging.[5,6] The Bohler angle can be used to access the degree of initial injury and severity of the fracture but is not usually used in evaluating postoperative fracture reduction. Postoperative fracture reduction should focus on the articular joint congruency surface along with reconstruction of the calcaneal body. The Bohler angle on initial presentation of less than 0° was associated with a significant increase of patients that will require a secondary subtalar joint arthrodesis. In addition, Sanders type 4 fractures are associated with a poor functional outcome after open reduction and internal fixation and a high incidence of secondary subtalar joint arthrodesis; therefore, primary arthrodesis has been advocated despite the surgical challenge (**Fig. 4**).

The most common constant fragment in displaced intra-articular calcaneal fractures is the sustentacular fragment and operative treatment typically consisted of a lateral approach, with the subtalar joint being reconstructed back to the sustentaculum tali. Reduction of the sustentaculum tali is achieved by anatomic reduction of the primary fracture line and medial wall. A medial approach is typically required when the sustentaculum tali is fractured and gapped from the posterior medial articular portion of the posterior facet. However, in a study by Berberian and colleagues,[7] after CT review of 100 displaced intra-articular calcaneal fractures, it was found that the sustentacular fragment was displaced in 42 fractures and more common with the 3- and 4-part calcaneal fractures.

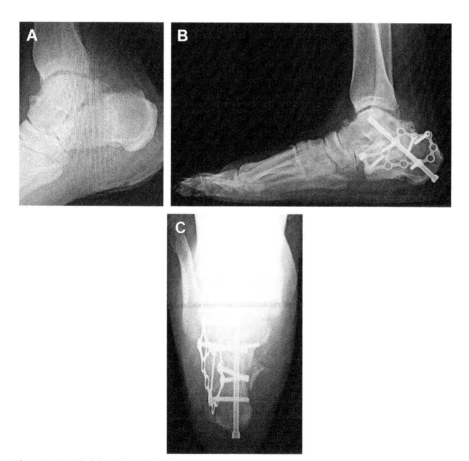

Fig. 4. Lateral (*A*) radiograph demonstrating an intra-articular joint-depressed calcaneal fracture. Lateral (*B*) and calcaneal axial (*C*) radiographs postoperatively demonstrating a primary subtalar joint arthrodesis with open reduction and internal fixation of the calcaneus.

SUMMARY

The surgical treatment of intra-articular calcaneal fractures requires understanding and a thorough evaluation of the fracture pattern and patient characteristics that may compromise the surgical outcome. An appropriate surgical approach is an important factor in obtaining a patient's successful outcome.

REFERENCES

1. Sagray BA, Stapleton JJ, Zgonis T. Diabetic calcaneal fractures. Clin Podiatr Med Surg 2013;30:111–8.
2. Facaros Z, Ramanujam CL, Zgonis T. Primary subtalar joint arthrodesis with internal and external fixation for the repair of a diabetic comminuted calcaneal fracture. Clin Podiatr Med Surg 2011;28:203–9.
3. Fu TH, Liu HC, Su YS, et al. Treatment of displaced intra-articular calcaneal fractures with combined transarticular external fixation and minimal internal fixation. Foot Ankle Int 2013;34:91–8.
4. Savva N, Saxby TS. In situ arthrodesis with lateral-wall ostectomy for the sequelae of fracture of the os calcis. J Bone Joint Surg Br 2007;89:919–24.
5. Su Y, Chen W, Zhang T, et al. Bohler's angle's role in assessing the injury severity and functional outcome of internal fixation for displaced intra-articular calcaneal fractures: a retrospective study. BMC Surg 2013;13:40.
6. Sanders R, Fortin P, DiPasquale T, et al. Operative treatment in 120 displaced intraarticular calcaneal fractures. Results using a prognostic computed tomography classification. Clin Orthop Relat Res 1993;290:87–95.
7. Berberian W, Sood A, Karanfilian B, et al. Displacement of the sustentacular fragment in intra-articular calcaneal fractures. J Bone Joint Surg Am 2013;95:995–1000.

Surgical Treatment of Tibial Plafond Fractures

John J. Stapleton, DPM[a,b,*], Thomas Zgonis, DPM[c]

KEYWORDS

- Tibial plafond fractures • Pilon fractures • Internal fixation • External fixation
- Surgery • Reconstruction

KEY POINTS

- Rotational distal tibial plafond fractures are usually associated with low-energy injuries.
- High-energy axial load injuries can result in tibial pilon fractures with severe intra-articular impaction, comminution of the metaphysis, and poor soft tissue envelope.
- Understanding the mechanism of injury, fracture pattern, and soft tissue injury is paramount to the patient's overall successful outcome.
- Open pilon fractures are surgically addressed in staged procedures with a thorough understanding of the role of free tissue transfer for major soft tissue defects.

INITIAL CARE PLAN

Ultimate success to the management of tibial plafond fractures stems from a logical systematic approach that is predicated on the overall assessment of the patient, fracture pattern, and associated soft tissue injury. Addressing the associated soft tissue injuries encountered with the tibia plafond fractures is paramount to the overall patient's successful outcome. Crushing injuries, open wounds, fracture blisters, and/or compartment syndrome are typically associated with the high-energy tibial plafond fractures. The surgical plan will need to be formulated early on at the initial presentation to determine whether a single or multiple staged procedures are required to achieve the definitive fracture reduction.

Tibial plafond fractures are often present among polytrauma patients with several body injuries. Although life-threatening trauma is a priority, the lower extremity needs

Disclosures: None.
[a] Foot and Ankle Surgery, VSAS Orthopaedics, Lehigh Valley Hospital, 1250 South Cedar Crest Boulevard, Suite # 110, Allentown, PA 18103, USA; [b] Penn State College of Medicine, 500 University Drive, Hershey, PA 17033, USA; [c] Reconstructive Foot and Ankle Surgery, Division of Podiatric Medicine and Surgery, Department of Orthopaedic Surgery, University of Texas Health Science Center San Antonio, 7703 Floyd Curl Drive MSC 7776, San Antonio, TX 78229, USA
* Corresponding author. Foot and Ankle Surgery, VSAS Orthopaedics, Podiatric Surgery, Lehigh Valley Hospital, 1250 South Cedar Crest Boulevard, Suite # 110, Allentown, PA 18103.
E-mail address: jostaple@hotmail.com

Clin Podiatr Med Surg 31 (2014) 547–564
http://dx.doi.org/10.1016/j.cpm.2014.06.002
0891-8422/14/$ – see front matter © 2014 Elsevier Inc. All rights reserved.

to be assessed to determine if early care is required for stabilization in a temporary and expedited fashion. Fractures with severe instability, open fractures, and fractures associated with compartment syndrome may need to be addressed in an expedited manner and if the patient's general condition permits. Open wounds should be meticulously debrided and irrigated to prevent septic complications; fasciotomies should be performed for the compartment syndrome, and unstable fractures may need to be stabilized with spanning external fixators. Closed fractures that are stable may be managed with an early application of well-padded splints and until a definitive surgical treatment plan can be performed. A simple bar to clamp external fixators is most commonly used in these types of injuries because they provide reliable temporary fracture stabilization in an expedited manner until the definitive surgical treatment is performed.

STEPWISE APPROACH

Single-staged procedures are reserved for low-energy rotational tibial plafond fractures without soft tissue compromise and relatively healthy individuals. These fractures are typically associated with little impaction of the articular surface and involve large fracture fragments that make reduction feasible through a limited approach and/or percutaneous plating (**Fig. 1**). Typically, the fibular fractures encountered along with the rotational tibial plafond fractures are fixated first, while the tibia can be fixated by means of a limited open reduction and internal fixation (ORIF), percutaneous plating, or standard ORIF of the tibia.[1] High-energy axial loading tibial plafond fractures are definitively fixated once the soft tissue envelope permits.[2]

Understanding the fracture pattern and forces that led to failure of the tibia are paramount in formulating a surgical approach. The AO/OTA (Arbeitsgemeinschaft für Osteosynthesefragen/Orthopaedic Trauma Association) classification system simplifies tibial plafond fractures into 3 broad categories with 3 subdivisions. Type A is extra-articular and is further divided into: A1: pure distal tibia metaphyseal fracture; A2: distal tibia metaphyseal wedge; and A3: complex distal tibia metaphyseal complex. Type B fracture is partially articular and is further divided into: B1: pure lateral split; B2: medial split with joint depression; and B3: posterior split with multiple fragmentary joint depression. Last, type C fractures are completely articular and are divided into: C1: articular fracture simple with metaphyseal fracture simple; C2: articular fracture simple with metaphyseal multifragmentary fracture; and C3: articular fracture multifragmentary with metaphyseal multifragmentary fracture.[3]

An associated tibia deformity with a varus or valgus component will alter the surgical approach and/or surgical construct to stabilize the tibia plafond. For example, a varus failure of the tibia is best treated with a medial buttress plate once the articular segment is secured (**Fig. 2**). On the other hand, a valgus failure of the tibia is better treated with an anterior-lateral plate. These basic principles of fixation will aid in neutralizing the major deforming forces that occur at the metaphyseal-diaphyseal junction and may prevent the incidence of hardware failure, malunion, and/or nonunion.

Preoperative planning is an essential part of the treatment of tibial plafond fractures. Careful evaluation of the preoperative radiographs will need to be compared and correlated with computed tomographic (CT) images to identify the individual fracture fragments that are amenable to reduction and those that need to be manipulated to gain access to areas of comminution. In many cases of high-energy and/or open tibia plafond fractures, the application of a spanning external fixator may need to be

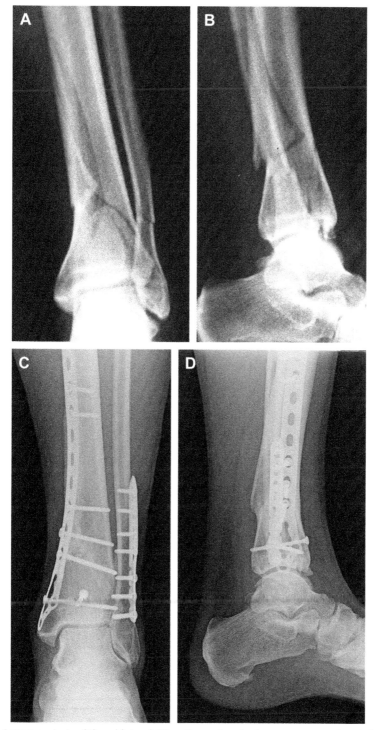

Fig. 1. Anteroposterior (*A*) and lateral (*B*) radiographs of a low-energy rotational tibia and fibula pilon fracture. Postoperative anteroposterior (*C*) and lateral (*D*) radiographs demonstrate reduction of the associated fractures. The fibula was fixated using a posterior lateral incision, while the tibia was fixated through a limited open reduction and percutaneous plate fixation in a single stage reconstruction.

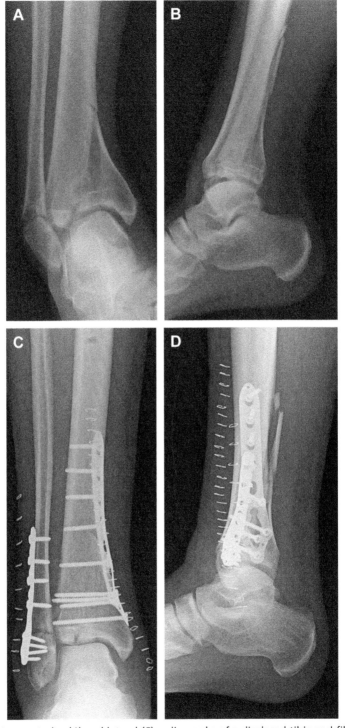

Fig. 2. Anteroposterior (*A*) and lateral (*B*) radiographs of a displaced tibia and fibula pilon fracture with varus deformity. Anteroposterior (*C*) and lateral (*D*) radiographs demonstrate an ORIF of the tibia pilon fracture with a medial buttress plate to neutralize the varus deformity. Definitive fixation of the tibia was performed 7 days after the initial ORIF of the fibula with a spanning external fixator.

performed in an expedited manner and before the CT imaging of the lower extremity. In those cases, CT imaging after the application of an external fixator provides a clinical benefit in regard to assessment of the fracture pattern and surgical approach to achieve definitive reduction. Obtaining CT scans for a grossly displaced tibia plafond fracture before the initial reduction will many times offer little information in regard to orientation of the fracture fragments and surgical approach.

FRACTURE PATTERN AND REDUCTION TECHNIQUES

OTA type A fractures require reduction of the tibial diaphysis to the articular segments. Emphasis is placed on applying internal plate fixation that counteracts with the deforming force of the tibia. Concomitant comminuted metaphyseal segments are associated with higher nonunion rates. Bone defects can be managed with simultaneous autogenous bone grafting versus placement of antibiotic cemented spacers and delayed autogenous bone grafting. In addition, plate osteosynthesis for these fractures should provide adequate stability and compression. OTA type B and C fractures often display significant impaction of the articular osteochondral surface. Understanding the common fracture fragments that are present on the articular surface is important in achieving a congruency of the articular joint.

The most common fracture fragments encountered are the posterior-lateral, anterior-lateral, medial, and central impaction (**Fig. 3**). The posterior-lateral fracture fragment is the essential fracture fragment to reduce first as the remainder of the articular reduction is fixated to the posterior-lateral fracture fragment. Larger posterior-lateral fragments are more amenable to plate fixation across the tibial metaphyseal-diaphyseal junction. Difficulty arises among smaller and significantly displaced posterior-lateral fracture fragments. Often, the ligamentous structures of the ankle remain intact after tibial plafond fractures and reduction of the posterior-lateral fracture fragment can be achieved through anatomic reduction of the fibula. Reduction can be carried out either through a posterior-lateral approach or by reflection of the anterior-lateral fragment and reduction by placement of a large pin fixation or curved periosteal elevator. Once the posterior-lateral fragment is reduced, the medial fragment is reduced and stabilized to the posterior-lateral fragment. The central impaction can then be addressed and stabilized followed by reduction of the anterior-lateral segment. Initially, reduction is performed with the placement of multiple Kirschner wires. Once the articular surface is congruent, Kirschner wires can be exchanged for screw fixation. Once reduction of the articular segment is achieved, plate osteosynthesis can be applied to secure the articular segment to the diaphysis. Additional reduction of the metaphysis and diaphysis can be performed with lag screws as necessary.

In certain cases, multiplane circular external fixators can be useful to achieve axial alignment and osseous union by avoiding fixation constructs that would interfere with eventual ankle arthrodesis (**Fig. 4**). Other options consist of a primary ankle arthrodesis with bone grafting using a blade plate or intramedullary nail. A circular external fixator can be used or combined with a blade plate and/or intramedullary nail if a primary ankle arthrodesis is performed.[4]

Open pilon fractures with extensive soft tissue loss require staged osteosynthesis with planned free tissue transfer. In addition, delayed autogenous bone grafting is often required to achieve union. In some cases, a proximal leg amputation may be indicated among these devastating injuries especially if neurovascular injury is evident in the presence of significant comminution, bone loss, and extensive soft tissue injury.

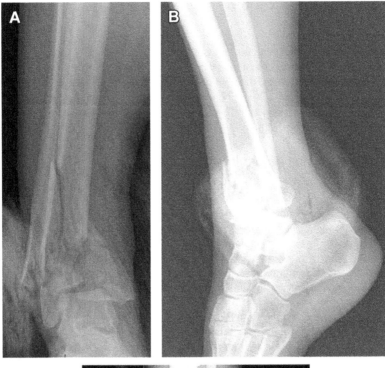

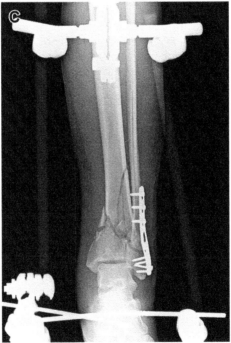

Fig. 3. Anteroposterior (*A*) and lateral (*B*) radiographs of a severely comminuted tibia pilon fracture. Note the common fracture fragments encountered consist of the anterolateral, posterolateral, medial fragment, and central comminution. This fracture pattern was also associated with a comminuted fracture involving the tibial metaphysis. Anteroposterior (*C*) postoperative radiograph demonstrates an ORIF of the fibula with spanning external fixation of the tibia. Postoperative long-term anteroposterior (*D*) and lateral (*E*) radiographs demonstrate successful union with posttraumatic arthritis of the ankle.

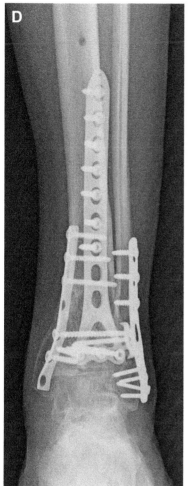
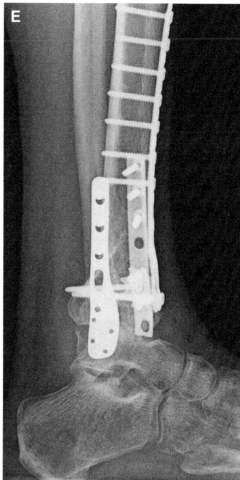

Fig. 3. (*continued*)

SURGICAL INCISIONAL APPROACHES
Anteromedial

The most common exposure to the tibial plafond fractures is an anteromedial approach. The traditional anteromedial approach allows for excellent exposure and visualization of the anterior and medial aspects of the plafond with limited lateral exposure unless the incision is slightly modified. Typically, the traditional incision is started 1 to 1.5 cm lateral to the anterior crest of the tibia and over the anterior compartment and fashioned distally to travel just medial to the tibialis anterior tendon. A full-thickness skin and subcutaneous tissue flap is elevated until the anterior tibial tendon is encountered. The extensor retinaculum and periosteum just medial to the anterior tibial tendon is then incised. A full-thickness flap that includes the skin, subcutaneous, and periosteal tissue is then elevated from the distal tibial metaphyseal region. Elevation of the anterior compartment allows for better access to the lateral aspect of the tibia. A longitudinal arthrotomy is performed at the interval of the main fracture split of the anterior tibial plafond and is extended to the level of the talar head. If an external

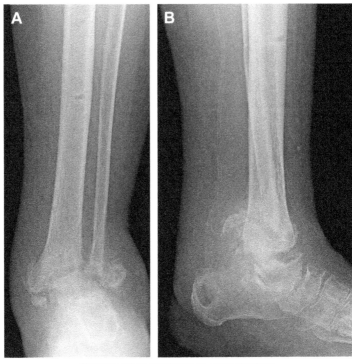

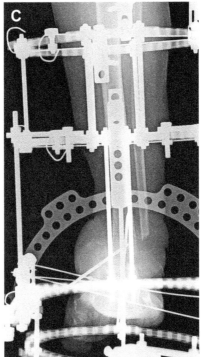

Fig. 4. Anteroposterior (*A*) and lateral (*B*) radiographs of a closed tibial plafond fracture in a patient with diabetic neuropathy with uncontrolled diabetes with peripheral arterial disease and multiple medical comorbidities. Primary tibiotalocalcaneal arthrodesis was performed with a multiplane circular external fixator (*C*, *D*). Postoperative long-term anteroposterior (*E*) and lateral (*F*) radiographs demonstrate successful fusion.

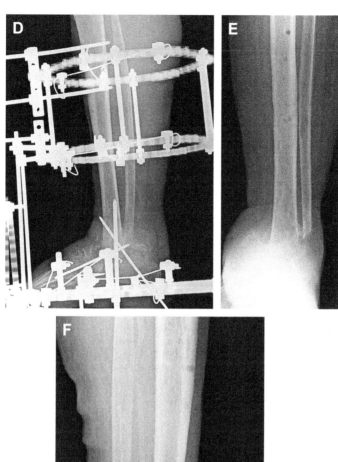

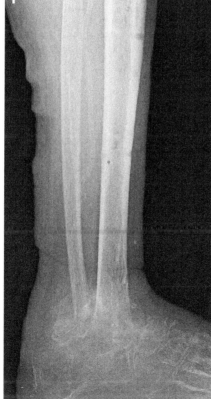

Fig. 4. (*continued*)

fixator was initially used to span the ankle joint, it can be reassembled to maintain distraction across the ankle to facilitate fracture reduction. Often, if a spanning external fixator was applied to initially stabilize the tibial plafond, the bars are disassembled before preparing the lower extremity, but the transcalcaneal and proximal half pins are not removed to allow reassembly of the spanning bars to serve as a distractor intraoperatively. If an external fixator was not initially used for a temporary fixation, a femoral/universal distractor can then be applied by placing a 4-mm Schantz pin into the medial aspect of the talar neck under direct visualization. An additional Schantz pin is then placed into the medial aspect of the proximal tibia diaphysis to allow for necessary distraction.

Anterolateral

The anterolateral approach is performed through an incision over the anterior lateral aspect of the ankle joint in alignment with the fourth metatarsal. After the skin incision is performed, the superficial peroneal nerve is identified and retracted medially. The extensor retinaculum and the fascia to the anterior compartment are then incised and the anterior compartment is raised and retracted medially. A longitudinal arthrotomy is made along the medial edge of the anterior-lateral (Chaput) fracture fragment (**Fig. 5**). This surgical exposure is advantageous to address any valgus angulation, significantly displaced Chaput fracture fragments, displaced posterior-lateral (Volkmann) and centrally impacted tibial plafond fracture fragments.[5] Limitations of the anterolateral approach are poor visualization of the medial tibial plafond and placement of internal fixation of the medial aspect of the distal tibia. Often, percutaneous plates can be placed medially if required. The anterolateral approach should be avoided for varus angulation and impaction of the medial tibial plafond. In addition, the skin bridge of an anterolateral approach if the fibula was fixated needs to be considered to avoid skin necrosis. Often, the fibula is fixated first through a posterior lateral incision followed by delayed fixation through an anterolateral incision that can be performed at a later stage and when the soft tissue envelope permits.

Direct Lateral Approach

The direct lateral approach to both the distal tibial plafond and the fibula is performed through a single incision fashioned over the fibula and extended distally in a curvilinear fashion at the tip of the fibula to the anterior process of the calcaneus. Dissection is carried down between the interval of the lateral and anterior compartments. Identification of the superficial peroneal nerve in the subcutaneous tissue is required and usually raised with the anterior compartment. The anterior compartment is raised with an intact soft tissue envelope of the tibia with blunt dissection preserving the angiosome of the anterior tibial artery. The ankle joint is exposed through a lateral longitudinal arthrotomy that is extended to the talar neck. This surgical incisional approach offers many advantages because a single incision is used, can provide access to concomitant comminuted fibula fractures associated with displaced lateral tibial plafond fractures, allows for direct visualization and reduction of valgus deformities of the tibial plafond with anterolateral plating, and, last, its exposure over the anterior compartment provides excellent soft tissue coverage over the bone and hardware.[6] Some limitations of this incision include its minimal exposure of the medial aspect of the tibial plafond. Medial malleolar fractures can be visualized and percutaneous screws can be placed, but difficulty would arise with more comminuted or impacted medial tibial plafond fractures such as those with an associated varus deformity. This direct lateral approach is usually advantageous for staged reconstruction of open pilon fractures that are associated with a medial wound and valgus deformity of the tibia.

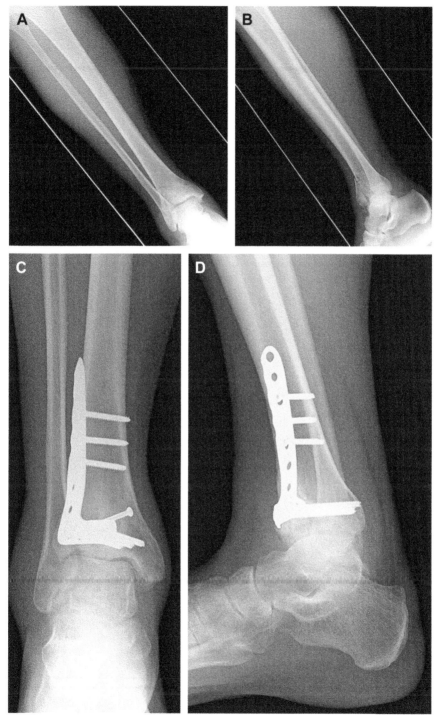

Fig. 5. Anteroposterior (*A*) and lateral (*B*) radiographs demonstrate a displaced tibial anterolateral "Chaput" fracture fragment with central impaction. Postoperative anteroposterior (*C*) and lateral (*D*) radiographs demonstrate an ORIF of the distal tibia through an anterolateral surgical exposure.

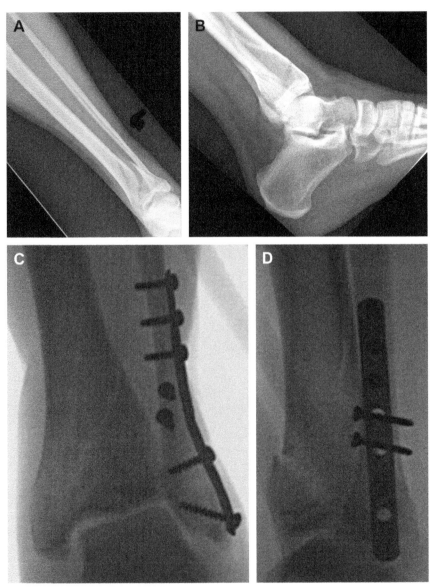

Fig. 6. Anteroposterior (*A*) and lateral (*B*) radiographs of a displaced tibia and fibula pilon fracture. C-arm fluoroscopy anteroposterior (*C*) and lateral (*D*) views after osteosynthesis of the fibula. Note the near anatomic reduction of the tibia secondary to ligamentotaxis. Postoperative long-term anteroposterior (*E*) and lateral (*F*) radiographs of the same injury after definitive ORIF of the tibia.

OSTEOSYNTHESIS OF THE FIBULA

A common surgical approach to staging tibial plafond fractures is to perform an ORIF of the fibula at the time the spanning external fixator is applied. The decision to address the fibula during the initial stage along with the application of a spanning

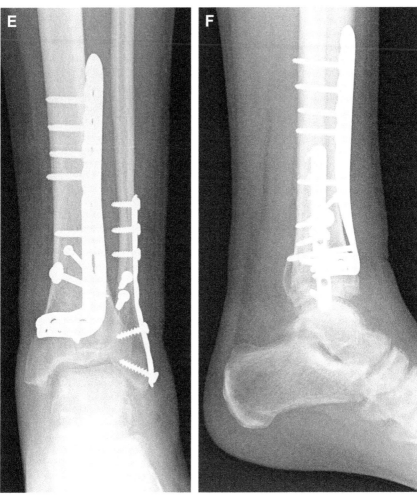

Fig. 6. (*continued*)

external fixator should be considered on the fracture pattern of the tibia, whether the fibula fracture is simple or complex, and the staged incisional placement that will be required to achieve definitive reduction of the tibial plafond. Fixation of the fibula is an important part of the initial reduction of tibia plafond fractures. Fibula fractures along with tibia plafond fractures differ in their fracture pattern when compared with low-energy rotational ankle fractures. If the fibula is fractured along with the tibia plafond fracture, they typically present in a comminuted, transverse, or oblique fracture pattern. Bone loss and mal-rotation are commonly encountered. For this reason, reduction needs to focus on providing stable constructs that allow restoration of fibula length, axial alignment, and rotation. Small fragment reconstruction plates, stacked one-third tubular plates, and/or dynamic compression plates for complex fibula shaft fractures are rigid and provide more stability versus one-third tubular plates that are commonly used for low-energy rotational lateral malleolar ankle fractures. Fixation

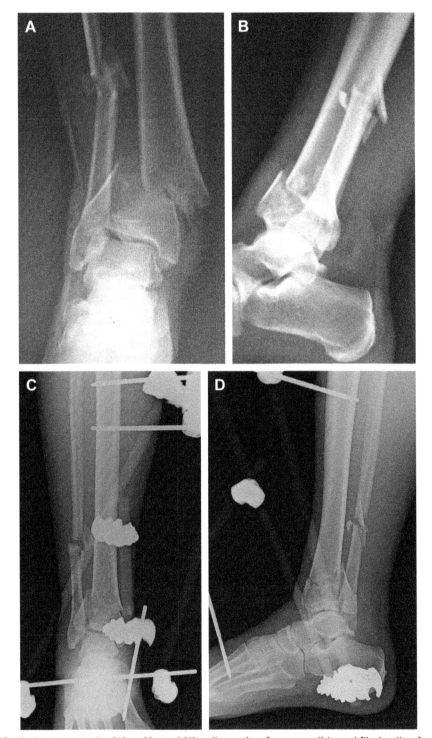

Fig. 7. Anteroposterior (*A*) and lateral (*B*) radiographs of an open tibia and fibula pilon fracture. Anteroposterior (*C*) and lateral (*D*) radiographs after surgical debridement of the open fracture and spanning external fixation. Postoperative anteroposterior (*E*) and lateral (*F*) radiographs of the fibula shaft and tibial plafond fracture fixated through a direct lateral approach. The tibia was fixated first given the degree of fracture comminution and bone loss noted to the fibula.

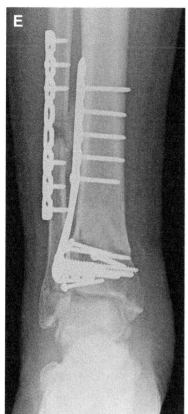
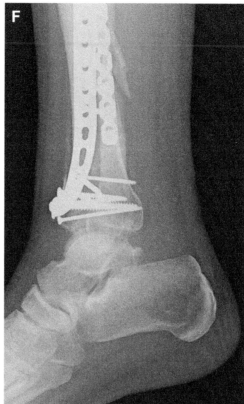

Fig. 7. (*continued*)

of simple fracture patterns of the fibula will provide reduction of most of the tibia pla-fond deformity secondary to the remaining ligamentous attachments (**Fig. 6**).

Fibular reduction is also beneficial to counteract significant valgus angulation and/or lateral translation of the tibia. However, in certain tibia plafond fractures that display significant valgus angulation with a concomitant comminuted fibula shaft fracture, a single direct lateral approach to address both the tibia and the fibula in one surgical setting may be at times advantageous. In open fractures with the aforementioned pattern, initial debridement of the open fracture and spanning external fixation is applied, while the tibia and fibula can be fixated through a single extensile lateral inci-sion in staged fashion. In addition, complex fibula fractures are preferably addressed after reconstruction of the tibia (**Fig. 7**). The syndesmosis ligamentous structures are usually intact, and therefore, realignment of the fibula occurs with reduction of the tibia, especially of the anterior-lateral and posterior-lateral fracture fragments of the tibia. Although reduction and stabilization of the fibula are important parts in the man-agement of tibia plafond fractures, careful consideration is given to the staged surgical approach for definitive fixation and before proceeding with fixation of the fibula during the initial surgical stage.

562

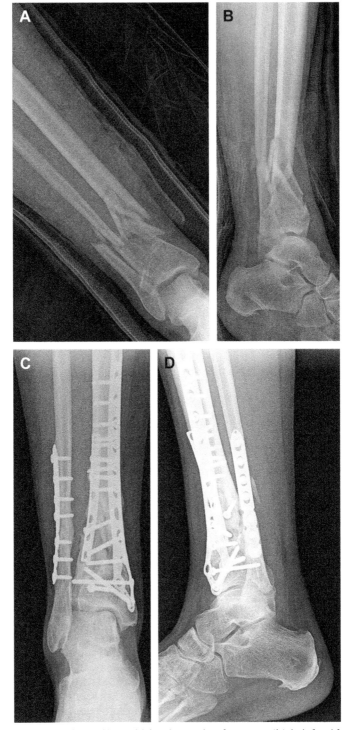

Fig. 8. Anteroposterior (*A*) and lateral (*B*) radiographs of an open tibial plafond fracture with significant comminution of the tibial metaphyseal-diaphyseal region. Postoperative long-term radiographs (*C*, *D*) show the nonunion of the metaphyseal-diaphyseal segment of the tibia, which was also confirmed with CT. Final anteroposterior (*E*) and lateral (*F*) radiographs demonstrate successful union with autogenous bone grafting to repair the tibia nonunion.

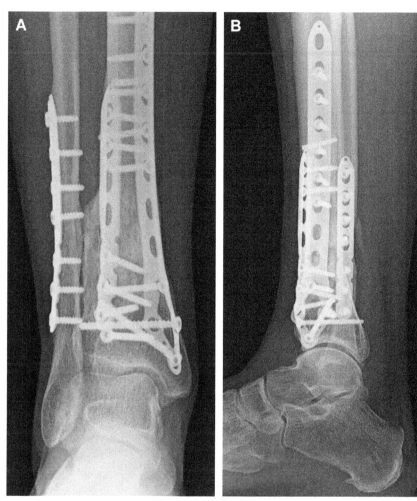

Fig. 8. (*continued*)

POSTOPERATIVE COMPLICATIONS

Although tibial plafond fractures are associated with many potential complications, those that require further surgery are the most challenging. Subsequent surgery may be required for wound-healing complications, infection, malunion, nonunion, and posttraumatic arthritis.[2,7] Prompt attention to infected wounds and/or osteomye-litis with meticulous debridement is paramount to promote healing. Wounds with exposed bone and/or hardware may require hardware removal and excision of all infected nonviable bone and soft tissue to provide a wound bed amenable to plastic surgery reconstruction. Bone transport, autogenous bone grafting, realignment osteotomies, and/or ankle arthrodesis may be necessary for the postoperative man-agement of tibial plafond complications (**Fig. 8**).

SUMMARY

The treatment necessary for tibial plafond fractures is best determined on an individual basis. Tibial plafond fractures and associated soft tissue injuries can be quite challenging to the surgeon, and careful attention is paid to the initial injury as well as the entire thought process of staged reconstruction when necessary. Treating these injuries in an efficient and expedited manner can prevent frequent complications encountered in this patient population.

REFERENCES

1. Davidovitch RI, Elkhechen RJ, Romo S, et al. Open reduction with internal fixation versus limited internal fixation and external fixation for high grade pilon fractures (OTA type 43C). Foot Ankle Int 2011;32:955–61.
2. Sirkin M, Sanders R, DiPasquale T, et al. A staged protocol for soft tissue management in the treatment of complex pilon fractures. J Orthop Trauma 2004;18: S32–8.
3. Orthopaedic Trauma Association Committee for Coding and Classification. Fracture and dislocation compendium. J Orthop Trauma 1996;10:56–60.
4. Lovisetti G, Agus MA, Pace F, et al. Management of distal tibial intra-articular fractures with circular external fixation. Strategies Trauma Limb Reconstr 2009;4:1–6.
5. Mehta S, Gardner MJ, Barei DP, et al. Reduction strategies through the anterolateral exposure for fixation of type B and C pilon fractures. J Orthop Trauma 2011; 25:116–22.
6. Femino JE, Vaseenon T. The direct lateral approach to the distal tibia and fibula: a single incision technique for distal tibial and pilon fractures. Iowa Orthop J 2009; 29:143–8.
7. Zalavras CG, Patzakis MJ, Thordarson DB, et al. Infected fractures of the distal tibial metaphysis and plafond: achievement of limb salvage with free muscle flaps, bone grafting, and ankle fusion. Clin Orthop Relat Res 2004;427:57–62.

The Mangled Foot and Ankle
Soft Tissue Salvage Techniques

Geoffrey G. Hallock, MD[a,b],*

KEYWORDS

- Mangled foot and ankle • Soft tissue reconstruction • Free flap • Perforator flap

KEY POINTS

- The mangled foot and ankle may be defined as an injury to multiple organ systems, but a significant loss of soft tissues may be the major determinant as to whether the limb is retrievable.
- Wound preparation if salvage is attempted requires an orderly progression of fracture fixation, revascularization if needed, and then débridement of all nonviable tissues. Any attempt at soft tissue coverage must be delayed until this requisite débridement has been completed.
- Because multiple foot subunits are typically involved in the mangled injury, the resultant large defects may be best covered by a free tissue transfer.
- The decision to salvage the mangled foot and ankle must be a team effort from the beginning and should include the opinion of a reconstructive microsurgeon to decide if it is even possible to restore the missing soft tissues.

Just what qualifies to be called a mangled foot or ankle injury may be a point of conjecture, but usually there is little doubt when seen (**Fig. 1**). Purists consider this to have to be a multisystem injury where 3 of 4 major organ systems (integument, vascular, nerve, and bone) have been simultaneously violated.[1–3] Others have broadened this appellation to include severe injuries that have occurred to only 2 of these 4 organ systems, but soft tissue loss alone has been extensive, with the latter perhaps so defined if it spans more than a single foot subunit (**Fig. 2**).[2] If a mangled foot or ankle has no soft tissue component, then the need for coverage is not a concern and the remainder of this article becomes irrelevant—but that is rarely the case.

Financial Disclosure: None.

[a] Division of Plastic Surgery, Sacred Heart Hospital and Lehigh Valley Hospital, 1230 South Cedar Crest Boulevard, Suite 306, Allentown, PA 18103, USA; [b] St. Luke's Hospital, Bethlehem, PA, USA

* 1230 South Cedar Crest Boulevard, Suite 306, Allentown, PA 18103.

E-mail address: gghallock@hotmail.com

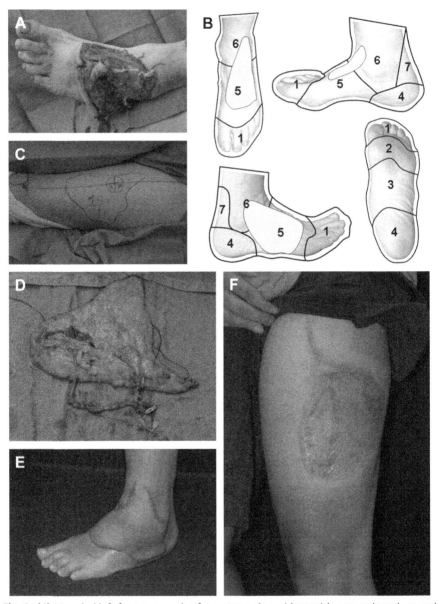

Fig. 1. (A) Mangled left foot as a result of a motor cycle accident with exposed tendons and extensive soft tissue loss, (B) involving subunits 5 and 6, (C) which required a megaflap for coverage, here designed as an ipsilateral anterolateral thigh (ALT) perforator flap about 2 perforators marked "x" found with an audible Doppler; (D) undersurface of ALT free flap with the 2 vastus lateralis musculocutaneous perforators on microgrid pieces that both joined the extremely long descending branch of the lateral circumflex femoral vessels vascular leash (in microclamp); (E) reasonable appearance and contour of the left foot required no secondary procedures; (F) because such a huge flap was necessary, a skin graft of the thigh donor site was needed to avoid a compartment syndrome.

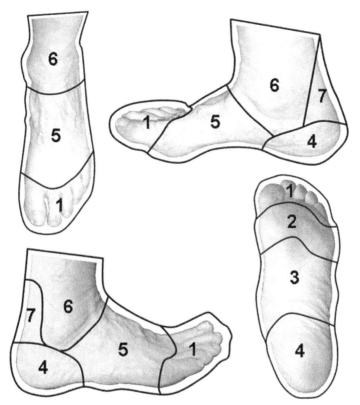

Fig. 2. Zones of the foot and ankle based on functional and aesthetic subunits (1, toes; 2, plantar forefoot; 3, plantar midfoot; 4, hindfoot; 5, dorsum of foot; 6, ankle joint and vicinity, encompassing medial and lateral malleoli; and 7, posterior hindfoot). (*Modified from* Hallock GG. Foot and ankle reconstruction. In: Blondeel PN, Morris SF, Hallock GG, et al, editors. Perforator flaps: anatomy, technique, & clinical applications, vol. 2. 2nd edition. St Louis (MO): Quality Medical Publishing; 2013. p. 1211.)

Homo sapiens is somewhat unique in the animal world in that they maintain an erect posture and simultaneously have mobilization capabilities that depend on the foot as a dynamic platform that must withstand constant load-bearing and shearing forces.[4] When confronted with a mangled foot or ankle, the initial treating surgical team must make the correct judgment to decide whether to proceed with an immediate amputation or begin the steps needed not only for salvage of the extremity but also the restoration of an adequate ambulatory function. This is never as simple as it seems, and several injury graded severity scores, such as Mangled Extremity Syndrome Index,[1] Mangled Extremity Severity Score,[5] Predictive Salvage Index,[2] and Limb Salvage Index,[2] have attempted to provide an objective mechanism for making this decision. Prospectively these have usually proved a futile exercise, because although adequate to decide when limb salvage should be undertaken, they are poor predictors of when amputation is more appropriate.[2,6–8] Although this debate is better discussed elsewhere in this entire issue, the easiest solution may not be the best long-term solution for a given individual. What can be more disastrous than Lange's[9] conundrum—"a protracted course of treatment resulting in a limb with minimal functional capability, or immediate amputation of a limb where reasonable functional potential was discarded?" If reasonable function cannot be expected, however, limb amputation should not be viewed as a failure but a respectable and definitive treatment option.[10,11]

Although most lower extremity injury graded severity scores were predicated on data based on tibial fractures alone,[1,2,5] the Lower Extremity Assessment Project (LEAP) also analyzed mangled foot and ankle cases where inclusion criteria was severe open hindfoot or midfoot injury that encompassed the presence of an insensate plantar surface, devascularization, a major degloving injury, or soft tissue injury requiring some form of coverage as well as Gustillo-Anderson grade IIIB open pilon or ankle fractures.[8] The LEAP study concluded that the severity of the soft tissue injury had the greatest impact on the decision to attempt limb salvage.[8] If true, whether or not a given soft tissue deficit can be restored at all becomes a factor of paramount importance that mandates that the judgment of a reconstructive microsurgeon be appropriately considered as part of an overall team effort that makes any final treatment decisions.

PREOPERATIVE ASSESSMENT
Non–Soft Tissue Issues

Other life-threatening injuries or comorbidities cannot be a concern and must rely on an accurate assessment by the trauma team that has been handling the initial patient presentation. If not contraindicated, soft tissue replacement then requires an orderly progression of interventions. Adequate fracture reduction by an orthopedic or podiatric surgeon must first be completed. Any vascular insufficiency must be rectified not only to sustain foot viability but also to retain the possibility of simpler local foot flaps for smaller wounds and potential vascular recipient sites if a free flap is essential.

Wound Preparation

It is next imperative that all devitalized tissue be removed even if structurally of some importance, because only a pristine wound avoids the risk of a later infection. Three words to remember how to accomplish this task are apropos—débridement, then débridement, and finally more débridement—until only viable tissues remain.[10] Many physicians assume that the now ubiquitous negative-pressure wound therapy devices alone suffice to accomplish this objective,[12] but there is never any substitute for a surgeon's touch.

There is no question that negative-pressure wound therapy devices reduce the needed frequency of dressing changes to thereby minimize patient discomfort, lessen the burden on the nursing staff, and prevent wound desiccation that occurs so often if conventional dressings are neglected.[13] This modality enhances the formation of granulation tissues and wound contraction by secondary intention that can result in spontaneous healing of a small defect or allow use of only an autogenous skin graft[14] or, if still unacceptable to complete closure, perhaps use of a bilaminar acellular dermal regeneration template.[15,16] For the sheer magnitude of the mangled foot and ankle defect, however, usually the negative-pressure wound therapy device must be realized as no more than a bridge to the definitive method for restoring skin integrity, and that for many of these wounds is preferably a free flap.[4,10]

Subunits

If a vascularized tissue transfer is imperative to provide bulk or cover exposed fractures, tendon, or neurovascular structures, as is inevitably the case with the mangled foot and ankle, it is important to review some basic concepts to insure an appropriate choice. Hidalgo and Shaw[17] and other investigators[18] have previously introduced the subunit principle that has divided the foot and ankle into discrete zones according to the specific unique tissue requirements for each (see **Fig. 2**, **Table 1**). For example, the highly specialized glabrous skin of the plantar surface of the foot is difficult to replace with a durable yet thin flap.[19] The dorsum of the foot must also be thin, but because highly visible, a final acceptable aesthetic appearance is of significant importance. This is also true for the ankle, but any impediment of motion is a functional concern. The Duke group has updated this important idea so that any flap selected must meet the functional and aesthetic demands of the given zone, with bulk or contour that does not impede the use of shoe wear and proper ambulation (see **Table 1**).[4]

The Duke group also listed their preferences for coverage for each foot and ankle zone,[4] which has been updated here to include perforator flaps that essentially are fasciocutaneous flaps that do not include muscle (**Table 2**).[10] Many flap donor sites that are adequate for a single subunit, as listed in **Table 2**, may not be able to provide enough surface area for the typical mangled foot and ankle deformity that by definition of the term involves 2 or more subunits simultaneously. For the same reason, local foot flaps[20,21] and distal-based neurocutaneous flaps[22] from the more proximal leg that have been championed as an alternative to microsurgical tissue transfers are inadequate. The cross-leg flap, as commonly used in the past century, would perhaps suffice as a desperation option,[23] but today is otherwise unacceptable in terms of the cost of long-term limb immobilization and need for a staged procedure.[19]

Timing

Although Godina[24] proselytized that any open lower extremity wound should be closed immediately or soon afterward, this is not usually logistically practical. Many investigators strongly believe that closure in the acute wound phase (ie, within the first week) is preferable, especially if bone, tendon, nerves, and vessels are exposed.[4] Not all wounds have the same characteristics, however, because more severe injuries may require more time than this before achieving a satisfactory mileau.[25] The negative-pressure wound therapy device has helped extend this window of opportunity to some degree but should not be considered a panacea without limit.[13] From a pragmatic standpoint, the sooner the better is a reasonable goal, because the inflammatory response and fibrosis of wound healing migrate from the wound of injury to encompass nearby possible recipient sites—making them more fragile, more difficult to dissect, more susceptible to vasospasm, and invariably the cause of microanastomotic nightmares.

Table 1
Flap attributes desirable for foot and ankle subunit soft tissue coverage

| Zone | Subunit | Requirements | | |
		Functional	Bulk	Aesthetics
1	Toes	None	Thin	Visible
2	Plantar forefoot	High demand: push-off point	Thin and durable	Minimal visibility
3	Plantar midfoot	None	Thin	Hidden
4	Hindfoot	High demand: weight bearing	Bulky and durable	Hidden
5	Dorsal foot	None	Thin	Highly visible
6	Ankle	Moderate: to allow motion	Thin and pliable	Some visibility
7	Posterior hindfoot	None	Thin	Some visibility

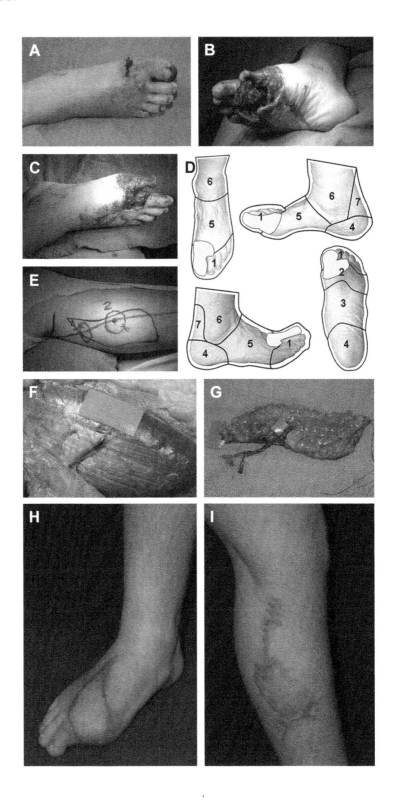

should not prevent simultaneous access to all foot subunits. In addition, either the anterior tibial or posterior tibial vessels can readily be exposed to serve as the requisite vascular recipient site. The vascular pedicle is long enough to usually allow reach outside the zone of injury without the need for vein grafts. The muscle is thin enough to replace any foot subunit, although atrophy and further thinning occur with time. Skin replacement requires a skin graft on the muscle, which is aesthetically displeasing.

It is always easier to maneuver within the operative theater when a patient is in a supine position. A perforator flap with characteristics similar to the subunit involved can be chosen specifically just for this reason. Patients cannot be morbidly obese because any donor site must be thin enough so that shoe wear can be worn during ambulation in an unimpeded fashion. As such, the medial sural artery perforator (MSAP) flap can be thin even in obese individuals (**Fig. 4**).[32] The MSAP flap can encompass almost all the skin of the calf and corresponds to the territory of the medial gastrocnemius muscle, because the latter's musculocutaneous perforator is its vascular source. This vascular leash has a length and caliber similar to those of the latissimus dorsi muscle. The donor site is nearby the foot and ankle defect so any iatrogenic morbidity is limited to the same lower extremity.[33] No muscle is included. No skin graft is needed so a reasonable aesthetic result is possible. A large flap requires a skin graft to close the donor site, however, and even direct closure leaves a vertical scar that is unacceptable, particularly for women.

Some reconstructive surgeons say that the anterolateral thigh perforator flap is the most ideal soft tissue flap of all (see **Fig. 1**).[34] Its surface area can exceed even that of the latissimus dorsi muscle. The potential vascular pedicle can be of large caliber and sometimes even too long, if that were possible. Again, the ipsilateral lower extremity can serve as the donor site to limit discomfort to the same leg. Fascia should not usually be included with the flap to maximize adherence to underlying structures during wound healing that minimizes wobbling during ambulation. A bulky flap in an obese patient is unacceptable for proper shoe fitting, so thinning might be needed primarily[35] or as a secondary procedure.[36] No skin graft is needed, but in a hirsute patient there is a contrast with the appearance of the rest of the foot. An exceedingly large flap also requires a donor site skin graft that is conspicuous.

Intraoperative Concerns

To reiterate, complete wound débridement must precede flap transfer. A template of the defect should be created to ascertain the dimensions and design of the chosen flap. Confirmation of an adequate vascular recipient site must be established prior to dividing the pedicle of the free flap. Flap harvest is followed by temporary exact insetting over the foot and ankle defect. Microanastomoses are then completed, usually in an end-to-side fashion for the artery to preserve all major leg source vessels to the foot, and end-to-end between flap vein(s) and deep venae comitantes adjacent to

◄───

Fig. 4. (A) Forklift crush injury with devascularization of left great toe region; (B) after débridement of all ischemic tissues, exposed proximal phalanx and first metatarsal phalangeal joint were preserved, (C) but with loss of surrounding skin, (D) involving subunits 1, 2, and 5; (E) design on medial ipsilateral calf of MSAP flap about 2 perforators "x" as ascertained with the audible Doppler; (F) subfascial course of central perforator kept with this flap seen emanating from medial head of the gastrocnemius muscle; (G) MSAP flap free on the back table, with microgrid under the perforators and microclamp on the relatively long medial sural vascular pedicle; (H) durable, thin soft tissue coverage of the medial foot; (I) large width of this flap required a donor site skin graft, which demonstrates a nonaesthetic compromise.

the arterial anastomosis, although superficial foot veins may be preferable if a larger caliber is needed. When flow is reestablished, permanent flap insetting is finished.

POSTOPERATIVE EXPECTATIONS

Unfortunately, a liability with free flaps is that the job is not yet done. Postoperative monitoring is essential because 95% of anastomotic catastrophies occur within the first 3 days.[37] Dangling and walking protocols after that depend on the extent of other bodily system involvements. Edema management requires limb elevation for an indeterminate period. When later appropriate, use of shoe wear should be chosen so that constriction at the recipient site is avoided, and pressure on an insensate flap does no harm. The Duke group found that the mean time to unrestricted ambulation after a free flap was greater than 3 months.[4]

Long-term secondary procedures may require flap re-elevation, such as the need for bone grafts. Care must be taken while raising the flap to not compromise its circulation, which is far more facile a task if a perforator flap had been used. Not infrequently, flap contours need readjustment, especially to reduce bulk, which is often avoided by use of a muscle flap, which naturally atrophies. Instability of the flap, especially due to intrinsic mobility or wobble, is most common over the heel and a concern for both muscle and perforator flaps that may need correction.[4]

SUMMARY

The decision to salvage the mangled foot and ankle in lieu of amputation cannot be taken lightly by a team of responsible physicians. A typical reconstructive microsurgery consultant usually insists that any soft tissue defect can be covered. Yet each patient must still be treated as an individual, because no simple protocol has yet been devised that meets the physical, social, psychological, or perhaps today the economic needs of everyone. The ultimate goal after these devastating injuries is to maximize restoration of an individual's lifestyle with the best possible outcome, and that is the ability to ambulate as independently as possible.

ACKNOWLEDGEMENT

David C. Rice, BS, Physician Extender, Sacred Heart Hospital, Allentown, and St. Luke's Hospital, Bethlehem, Pennsylvania assisted with the operative procedures.

REFERENCES

1. Gregory RT, Gould RJ, Peclet M, et al. The mangled extremity syndrome (M.E.S.): a severity grading system for multisystem injury of the extremity. J Trauma 1985; 25:1147–50.
2. Bonanni F, Rhodes M, Lucke JF. The futility of predictive scoring of mangled lower extremities. J Trauma 1993;34:99–104.
3. de Mestral C, Sharma S, Haas B, et al. A contemporary analysis of the management of the mangled lower extremity. J Trauma Acute Care Surg 2013;74:597–603.
4. Medina ND, Kovach SJ III, Levin LS. An evidence-based approach to lower extremity acute trauma. Plast Reconstr Surg 2011;127:926–34.
5. Helfetm DL, Howeym T, Sandersm R, et al. Limb salvage versus amputation: preliminary results of the mangled extremity severity score. Clin Orthop Relat Res 1990;256:80–6.

6. Ly TV, Travison TG, Castillo RC, et al, LEAP Study Group. Ability of lower-extremity injury severity scores to predict functional outcome after limb salvage. J Bone Joint Surg Am 2008;90:1738–43.
7. Bosse MJ, MacKenzie EJ, Kellam JF, et al. A prospective evaluation of the clinical utility of the lower-extremity injury severity scores. J Bone Joint Surg Am 2001;83: 3–14.
8. Swiontkowski MF, MacKenzie EJ, Bosse MJ, et al, LEAP Study Group. Factors influencing the decision to amputate or reconstruct after high-energy lower extremity trauma. J Trauma 2002;52:641–9.
9. Lange RH. Limb reconstruction vs amputation decision making in massive lower extremity trauma. Clin Orthop 1989;243:92–9.
10. Hallock GG. Evidence-based medicine: lower extremity acute trauma. Plast Reconstr Surg 2013;132:1733–41.
11. Hallock GG. Utility of both muscle and fascia flaps in severe lower extremity trauma. J Trauma 2000;48:913–7.
12. Hallock GG. To VAC or not to VAC? Ann Plast Surg 2007;59:473–4.
13. Hou Z, Irgit K, Strohecker KA, et al. Delayed flap reconstruction with vacuum-assisted closure management of the open IIIb tibial fracture. J Trauma 2011; 71:1705–8.
14. Ullman Y, Fodor L, Ramon Y, et al. The revised reconstructive ladder and its applications for high-energy injuries to the extremities. Ann Plast Surg 2006;56: 401–5.
15. Ghazi BH, Williams JK. Use of integra in complex pediatric wounds. Ann Plast Surg 2011;66:493–6.
16. Park CA, Defranzo AJ, Marks MW, et al. Outpatient reconstruction using integra and subatmospheric pressure. Ann Plast Surg 2009;62:164–9.
17. Hidalgo DA, Shaw WW. Reconstruction of foot injuries. Clin Plast Surg 1986;13: 663–80.
18. Hallock GG. Cutaneous coverage for the difficult wound of the foot. Contemp Orthop 1988;16:19–30.
19. Hong JP, Kim EK. Sole reconstruction using anterolateral thigh perforator free flaps. Plast Reconstr Surg 2007;119:186–93.
20. Hallock GG. Local fasciocutaneous flap skin coverage for the dorsal foot and ankle. Foot Ankle 1991;11:275–81.
21. Hallock GG. Distally based flaps for skin coverage of the foot and ankle. Foot Ankle Int 1996;17:343–8.
22. Nakajima H, Imanishi N, Fukuzumi S, et al. Accompanying arteries of the cutaneous veins and cutaneous nerves in the extremities: anatomical study and a concept of the venoadipofascial and/or neuroadipofascial pedicled fasciocutaneous flap. Plast Reconstr Surg 1998;102:779–91.
23. Lu L, Liu A, Zhu L, et al. Cross-leg flaps: our preferred alternative to free flaps in the treatment of complex traumatic lower extremity wounds. J Am Coll Surg 2013; 217:461–71.
24. Godina M. Early microsurgical reconstruction of complex trauma of the extremities. Plast Reconstr Surg 1986;78:285–92.
25. Hutson JJ Jr, Dayicioglu D, Oeltjen JC, et al. The treatment of Gustilo grade IIIB tibia fractures with application of antibiotic spacer, flap, and sequential distraction osteogenesis. Ann Plast Surg 2010;64:541–52.
26. Santanelli F, Tenna S, Pace A, et al. Free flap reconstruction of the sole of the foot with or without sensory nerve coaptation. Plast Reconstr Surg 2002;109: 2314–22.

27. Bosse MJ, McCarthy ML, Jones AL, et al, Lower Extremity Assessment Project (LEAP) Study Group. The insensate foot following severe lower extremity trauma: an indication for amputation? J Bone Joint Surg Am 2005;87(A):2601–8.
28. Hallock GG. In an era of perforator flaps, are muscle flaps passe? Plast Reconstr Surg 2009;123:1357–63.
29. Hallock GG. If based on citation volume, perforator flaps have landed mainstream. Plast Reconstr Surg 2012;130:769e–71e.
30. Hallock GG. Foot and ankle reconstruction. In: Blondeel PN, Morris SF, Hallock GG, et al, editors. Perforator flaps: anatomy, technique, & clinical applications, vol. 2, 2nd edition. St Louis (MO): Quality Medical Publishing; 2013. p. 1209–22.
31. May JW Jr, Lukash FN, Gallico GG III. Latissimus dorsi free muscle flap in lower-extremity reconstruction. Plast Reconstr Surg 1981;68:603–7.
32. Hallock GG. The medial sural MEDIAL GASTROCNEMIUS perforator free flap: an 'ideal' prone position skin flap. Ann Plast Surg 2004;52:184–7.
33. Hallock GG. Medial sural artery perforator free flap: legitimate use as a solution for the ipsilateral distal lower extremity defect. J Reconstr Microsurg 2014;30(3):187–92. http://dx.doi.org/10.1055/s-0033-1357276.
34. Wei FC, Jain V, Celik N, et al. Have we found an ideal soft-tissue flap? an experience with 672 anterolateral thigh flaps. Plast Reconstr Surg 2002;109:2219–26.
35. Hong JP, Chung IW. The superficial fascia as a new plane of elevation for anterolateral thigh flaps. Ann Plast Surg 2013;70:192–5.
36. Hallock GG. Conventional liposuction-assisted debulking of muscle perforator flaps. Ann Plast Surg 2004;53:39–43.
37. Chen KT, Mardini S, Chuang DC, et al. Timing of presentation of the first signs of vascular compromise dictates the salvage outcome of free flap transfers. Plast Reconstr Surg 2007;120:187–95.

Strategies for Managing Bone Defects of the Lower Extremity

Vasilios D. Polyzois, MD, PhD*, Ioannis P. Stathopoulos, MD, MSc, Kalliopi Lampropoulou-Adamidou, MD, MSc, Elias S. Vasiliadis, MD, PhD, John Vlamis, MD, PhD, Spiros G. Pneumaticos, MD, PhD

KEYWORDS

- Induced membranes • RIA technique • Masquelet technique • Papineau technique
- Ilizarov technique • Distraction osteogenesis

KEY POINTS

- Cancellous autograft harvesting by Reamer irrigator aspirator (RIA) method for filling bone voids.
- Use of bone cement for development of induced membranes to later host cancellous autografts.
- Internal fixation and intramedullary nailing in combination with Masquelet technique.
- Papineau technique in combination with external fixation for dealing with composite bone and soft tissue loss.
- Ilizarov technique and distraction osteogenesis as method of choice in the management of combined bone and soft tissue loss.

Management of posttraumatic segmental bone loss as a result of severe open injuries of the lower extremity continues to challenge reconstructive surgeons. Surprisingly severe posttraumatic bone loss of the lower extremity can also occur after very high-energy closed injuries and certainly following failed initial treatment of complex fractures that develop pseudarthrosis, with or without septic complications.

The literature proposes numerous strategies for dealing with such injuries but it is clear that the outcome is often unpredictable. The procedure rarely involves only one stage and complications frequently arise. In most cases the reconstruction process is long and difficult and amputation must be part of the decision-making process in the first place and can be a possible outcome if the reconstructive procedure fails, even after great effort.

Disclosures: None.
3rd Department of Orthopaedics and Traumatology, KAT Hospital, 2 Nikis Street, Kifisia, Athens 14561, Greece
* Corresponding author.
E-mail address: vpolyzois@gmail.com

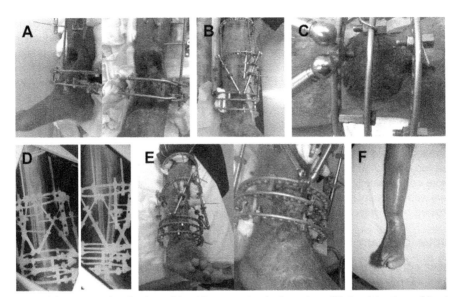

Fig. 1. (*A*) Major right tibial combined bone and soft tissue loss. (*B*) Combination of Papineau technique for the distal tibial injury and lengthening proximally. (*C*) The bulky mass of cancellous autografts that are left exposed. (*D*) Healing of both lengthening and Papineau sites. (*E*) Gradual "metaplasia" of the outer layer of the autografts. (*F*) Both bone and soft tissue loss healed out.

mesh cages in severe open type IIIb fractures, mostly after initial debridement and irrigation and a few by means of one-stage procedure with flap coverage. Because the cage cannot provide adequate stabilization alone, statically locked intramedullary nailing or plating was performed on top. There are no reports about septic complications despite the presence of massive implanted hardware in the previously injured extremity with soft tissue compromise.

POROUS TANTALUM CONES AND CYLINDERS

A new material has been introduced and reports about its efficiency were published during the last decades. The porous tantalum shaped as a rod was initially used for the management of avascular necrosis of the femoral head before its collapse stage and in the shape of cones for the management of large bone defects of the acetabulum and the proximal tibial metaphysis in revision total joint surgery, demonstrating excellent performance that encouraged other authors to extend its use in foot and ankle surgery. Porous tantalum recently has been used for rear foot and ankle arthrodesis when large bone defects are present.[12] Preliminary data suggest that porous tantalum may be used as a structural graft even in cases of traumatic bone loss of the lower extremity as long as adequate soft tissue coverage of the material can be reconstructed.

EXTERNAL FIXATION METHODS

External fixation methods have distinct advantages for the treatment of lower extremity bone loss, especially in infected cases. The so-called transosseous osteosynthesis as introduced by Ilizarov more than six decades ago offers the advantage of immediate functional use of the injured extremity. The method is actually an internal lengthening of a specific anatomic segment.[13] A corticotomy is required, and in many cases two or even three corticotomies are advised for the treatment of larger defects. The corticotomy not only allows transportation of a bone segment but also transports the soft tissues attached to the transported bone segment. In this way large soft tissue gaps can be addressed simultaneously with bone gaps. Large half pins are used when there is need for combined soft tissue transport because they apply more force than smooth wires that actually cut the skin and the underlying tissues. Moreover, the corticotomy is a powerful stimulus to increase the limb's blood supply with neovascularization.[14] The Ilizarov method is reported to have fewer failures and major complications, possibly because no internal fixation hardware is definitively attached to the host bone.[15] The Ilizarov apparatus and method can provide solutions in cases that cannot be addressed by other means, such as in recurrent infection and periarticular bone loss. The main problem with the technique is its long learning curve and the experience needed to confront various types of minor and moderate complications, such as pin site infections, deformity, deviation of transported segments, and impingement of device parts blocking the transporting procedure. The most difficult problem when performing a bone transport technique is to achieve union at the docking site of the transported segment. If the surgeon goes for preservation of the original length of the extremity and internal transportation of a bone segment, pseudarthrotic fibrous tissue eventually interposes when the segment reaches the docking point. This issue has to be treated as another atrophic nonunion. More autogenous bone graft has to be harvested and used and axial compression must be applied. Another critical issue is the osteogenetic response to the corticotomy. In general, a properly performed low-energy corticotomy with preservation of the periosteum is advised, whereas high-energy osteotomy, oscillating saws, and gigli saws must be avoided together with anti-inflammatory medication throughout the procedure. The surgeon must be alert for the possibility of poor bone formation and there are several things one can do if this actually happens. Percutaneous bone marrow injection is a safe and useful technique with or without autogenous bone graft.[16] With this technique a large number of pluripotent stem cells are harvested and injected under fluoroscopic control in the anatomic site of the corticotomy and regenerate bone. Very rarely, reversal of the internal lengthening procedure if no bone is apparent in the corticotomy site is advised.[17]

Various types of external fixation devices can be used for bone and soft tissue transport applications, with the traditional Ilizarov device being the most favorable option. Software-assisted cyclic fixators are becoming more popular. For the treatment of femoral bone loss rail-type monolaterals provide better "in frame" quality of life and have to be considered the fixator of choice, especially if the devices will be attached for a long period of time. The "in frame" duration of treatment is a very critical factor not only for the reconstructive procedure but for the patient's tolerance, psychological condition, and quality of life in general. The "transport over nail" technique significantly reduces this period because the external fixator stays in place only until the transported segments reach their docking positions and the intramedullary nail ensures the static fixation after the removal of the external device.[18] Another strategy for reducing the "in frame" period in the management of very large tibial osseous defects is the tibialization of the fibula. The technique of longitudinal corticotomy of the fibula is one option. It is a demanding procedure and special configuration of the external device is necessary with use of olive wires to transport the split inner portion of the fibula anteriorly and medially. This way a thick and rapidly healing iatrogenic tibiofibular synostosis is produced with a 4-cm anteromedial transportation of the split fibula (**Fig. 2**). Another option is to perform a transportation of the fibula without

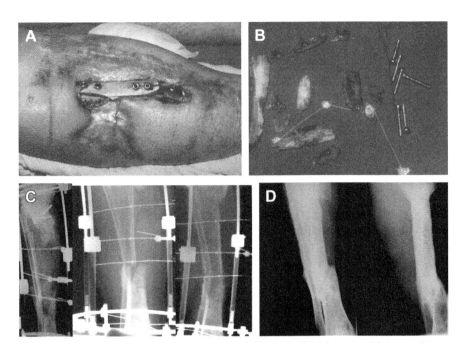

Fig. 2. (*A*) Failed internal fixator of comminuted midshaft tibial fracture. (*B*) Exposed internal fixation hardware and avascular tibial bone fragments resulting in major bone loss. (*C*) Longitudinal corticotomy of the fibula and anteromedial transportation of the inner portion of the fibula. (*D*) Tibialization of the fibula.

performing a splitting corticotomy but by performing a traditional horizontal osteotomy proximal to the bone's dominant vascular supply and dragging the distal part of the fibula anteromedially in site of the gap. Authors performing the last technique document that the transported fibula retains its vascular supply if the transport rhythm is low and also demonstrated hyperthrophy of the bone with gradual application of axial loading.[19,20]

VASCULARIZED FIBULAR TRANSPORT

Vascularized fibular transport is another option for the management of large defects, clean or infected, mostly of the tibia. The technique was first introduced for the management of avascular necrosis of the femoral head in early stages. It became popular in more fields of reconstructive surgery, such as management of posttraumatic osseous defects of the lower extremity. The main disadvantages of the technique are that it is demanding technically, donor site problems, inadequate hypertrophy of the graft, and occurrence of refractures when the protected weight-bearing period is over. These disadvantages did not allow this technique to dominate in lower extremity bone loss as it has succeeded in other fields, such as mandibular bone loss and upper extremity bone loss. The surgeon has two options for fixation of the free fibula within the bone gap: plating with screws or external fixation. Intramedullary nails cannot be introduced. The non–weight-bearing and protected weight-bearing periods are prolonged until radiographic evidence of secure union and hypertrophy of the graft are apparent. Efforts with the use of vascularized ribs or vascularized iliac crest have also been reported.[21–23]

SUMMARY

The Ilizarov technique is still considered as the treatment of choice having reproducibly good functional results and being the most versatile and applicable in all post-traumatic bone loss cases, minimizing the necessity for adjunctive therapies.[24,25] The recently revisited Papineau technique and the Masquelet/induced membrane technique are expanding their indications with the assistance of the RIA grafting method.[26,27] Tissue engineering is a new and developing option introduced to overcome limitations of bone grafts and improve the healing processes of bone fractures and defects. The combined use of ceramic or polymeric biomaterials as scaffolds, healing-promoting factors, gene therapy, and more recently three-dimensional printing of tissue-engineered constructs may open new insights in the near future.[28-30]

REFERENCES

1. Pneumaticos SG, Triantafyllopoulos GK, Basdra EK, et al. Segmental bone defects: from cellular and molecular pathways to the development of novel biological treatments. J Cell Mol Med 2010;14(11):2561-9.
2. van Winkle BA, Neustein J. Management of open fractures with sterilization of large, contaminated, extruded cortical fragment. Clin Orthop Relat Res 1987;(223):275-81.
3. Lerman OZ, Kovach SJ, Levin LS. The respective roles of plastic and orthopaedic surgery in limb salvage. Plast Reconstr Surg 2011;127(Suppl 1):215S-27S.
4. Giannoudis PV, Faour O, Goff T, et al. Masquelet technique for the treatment of bone defects: tips – tricks and future directions. Injury 2011;42(6):591-8.
5. Cuthbert RJ, Churchman SM, Tan HB, et al. Induced periosteum a complex cellular scaffold for the treatment of large bone defects. Bone 2013;57(2):484-92.
6. Koutsostathis SD, Lepetsos P, Polyzois VD, et al. Combined use of Ilizarov external fixation and Papineau technique for septic pseudarthrosis of the distal tibia in a patient with diabetes mellitus. Diabet Foot Ankle 2014;5. http://dx.doi.org/10.3402/dfa.v5.22841.
7. Karargyris O, Polyzois VD, Karabinas P, et al. Papineau debridement, Ilizarov bone transport and negative pressure wound closure for septic bone defects of the tibia. Eur J Orthop Surg Traumatol 2014;24(6):1013-7.
8. Polyzois VD, Galanakos SP, Tsiampa VA, et al. The use of Papineau technique for the treatment of diabetic and non-diabetic lower extremity pseudarthrosis and chronic osteomyelitis. Diabet Foot Ankle 2011;2. http://dx.doi.org/10.340/dfa.v2i0.5920.
9. Attias N, Lehman RF, Bodell LS, et al. Surgical management of a long segmental defect using a cylindrical titanium mesh cage and plates: a case report. J Orthop Trauma 2005;19(3):211-6.
10. Cobos JA, Lindsey RW, Gugala Z. The cylindrical titanium mesh cage for treatment of a long bone segmental defect: description of a new technique and report of two cases. J Orthop Trauma 2000;14(1):54-9.
11. Ostermann PA, Haase N, Rubberdt A, et al. Management of a long segmental defect at the proximal meta-diaphyseal junction of the tibia using a cylindrical titanium mesh cage. J Orthop Trauma 2002;16(8):597-601.
12. Frigg A, Dougall H, Boyd S, et al. Can porous tantalum be used to achieve ankle and sutalar arthrodesis? A pilot study. Clin Orthop Relat Res 2010;468(1):209-16.
13. Sala F, Thabet AM, Castelli F, et al. Bone transport for postinfectious segmental tibial bone defects with a combined Ilizarov/Taylor spatial frame technique. J Orthop Trauma 2011;25(3):162-8.

14. Brutscher R, Rahn BA, Ruter A, et al. The role of corticotomy and osteotomy in the treatment of bone defects using the Ilizarov technique. J Orthop Trauma 1993; 7(3):261–9.

15. Sella EJ. Prevention and management of complications of the Ilizarov treatment method. Foot Ankle Spec 2008;1(2):105–7.

16. Hatzokos I, Stavridis SI, Iosifidou E, et al. Autologous bone marrow grafting combined with demineralized bone matrix improves consolidation of the docking site after distraction osteogenesis. J Bone Joint Surg Am 2011;93(7):671–8.

17. Delloye C, Delefortrie G, Coutelier L, et al. Bone regenerate formation in cortical bone during distraction lengthening. An experimental study. Clin Orthop Relat Res 1990;(250):34–42.

18. Karargyris O, Romoudis P, Morassi LG, et al. Distraction over nail using circular external fixation for septic pseudarthrosis of the tibia. J Long Term Eff Med Implants 2012;22(2):137–43.

19. Shafi R, Fragomen AT, Rozbruch R. Ipsilateral fibular transport using Ilizarov–Taylor spatial frame for a limb salvage reconstruction: a case report. HSS J 2009;5(1):31–9.

20. Catagni MA, Ottaviani G, Camagni M. Treatment of massive tibial bone loss due to chronic draining osteomyelitis: fibula transport using the Ilizarov frame. Orthopedics 2007;30(8):608–11.

21. Yokohama K, Itoman M, Nakamura K, et al. Free vascularized fibular graft vs. Ilizarov method for post-traumatic tibial bone defect. J Reconstr Microsurg 2001; 17(1):17–25.

22. Amr SM, El Mofty AO, Amin SN. Anterior vs. posterior approach in reconstruction o infected nonunion of the tibia using the vascularized fibular graft: potentialities and limitations. Microsurgery 2002;22(3):91–107.

23. Legre R, Samson P, Tomei F, et al. Treatment of substance loss of the bones of the leg in trauamtology by transfer of the free vascularized iliac crest. Rev Chir Orthop Reparatrice Appar Mot 1998;84(3):264–71.

24. Kovoor CC, Padmanabhan V, Bhaskar D, et al. Ankle fusion for bone loss around the ankle joint using the Ilizarov technique. J Bone Joint Surg Br 2009;91(3): 361–6.

25. Rochman R, Jackson Hudson J, Alade O. Tibiocalcaneal arthrodesis using the Ilizarov technique in the presence of bone loss and infection of the talus. Foot Ankle Int 2008;29(10):1001–8.

26. Archdeacon MT, Messerschmitt P. Modern Papineau technique with vacuum-assisted closure. J Orthop Trauma 2006;20(2):134–7.

27. Taylor BC, French BG, Fowler TT, et al. Induced membrane technique for reconstruction to manage bone loss. J Am Acad Orthop Surg 2012;20(3):142–50.

28. Habibovic P, de Groot K. Osteoinductive biomaterials-properties and relevance in bone repair. J Tissue Eng Regen Med 2007;1(1):25–32.

29. Rai B, Oest ME, Dupont KM, et al. Combination of platelet-rich plasma with polycaprolactone-tricalcium phosphate scaffolds for segmental bone defect repair. J Biomed Mater Res 2007;81(4):888–99.

30. Oryan A, Alidadi S, Moshiri A, et al. Bone regenerative medicine: classic options, novel strategies and future directions. J Orthop Surg Res 2014;9(1):18.

Rehabilitation After Major Extremity Trauma

George F. Wallace, DPM, MBA

KEYWORDS

- Maximum medical improvement • Workman's compensation
- Foot and ankle trauma • Rehabilitation after foot and ankle trauma
- Independent medical examiner

KEY POINTS

- Physical therapy is an integral part of rehabilitation after foot and ankle trauma.
- Workman's compensation may play a role in treatment, prognosis, and added bureaucracy.
- The foot and ankle surgeon needs to be able to determine when maximum medical improvement has been reached.
- Patients with foot and ankle trauma must have a coordinated care plan, which may include a case manager, a physician conducting an independent medical examination, and possibly, legal counsel.

INTRODUCTION

Major traumas of the foot and ankle have been discussed in previous chapters of this issue. The first priority is to determine the mechanism of injury. In most instances, the injured foot and ankle patient is conscious and, despite pain, is able to relate just how the injury occurred. Then, we try to classify the injury; for example, using the Sanders' classification of calcaneal fractures.[1] The most complete classification provides treatment algorithms and prognosis.

During the course of treatment, physical therapy may be necessary to provide modalities to increase strength and range of motion and to decrease edema and pain. When to initiate this part of treatment is not necessarily clear-cut. The patient walks on the results, which can be a challenge to the physician and injured person.

Whether the patient with foot and ankle trauma walks into an office or is seen in the emergency room or trauma bay, it must be determined if the patient needs to be treated conservatively or with some form of invasive procedure. There may be many

---

Disclosures: none.
Podiatry Service, University Hospital, 150 Bergen Street, G-142, Newark, NJ 07103, USA
E-mail address: WALLACGF@UHNJ.org

comorbidities, with multiple pharmaceutical agents being taken. The patient must have the proper evaluation as to whether crutches and non–weight bearing are possible. Multiple specialties may be called, to ensure that the limb and the patient survive. In some instances, if a patient with similar comorbidities presented for hallux abductovalgus correction, you would forgo surgery. In trauma, this same patient would have to be medically optimized to repair the damage. Unable to use crutches? Maybe a wheelchair is prescribed. No help at home? Time spent in a subacute or rehabilitation facility would be arranged.

The patient may have been injured on the job. The injury may be so devastating and life altering that permanent disability results. The foot and ankle surgeon becomes a conduit to facilitate rehabilitation and to complete any steps necessary for applying for disability.

REHABILITATION

The goal, after injury, is to provide the patient with a stable plantigrade foot. Also included is the absence of pain, the ability to wear shoes even if prescribed (rocker soles, extra depth), or bracing a lower extremity. In some instances, when a toe(s), foot, or lower extremity is not salvageable, a prosthetic is necessary. A certified pedorthist/orthotist then becomes part of the team.[2]

One of the tenets of the Association for Osteosynthesis/Association for the Study of Internal Fixation is early mobilization and rehabilitation of the injured part and patient.[3] This tenet dovetails with anatomic reduction and stable fixation. Mobilization is important even if an invasive procedure was not performed.

Rehabilitation begins immediately after treatment. Rest, ice, compression, and elevation are instigated. The patient, depending on the injured part, may be prompted to move their toes or more proximal joints. Adequate pain control, using a standard pain protocol, patient-controlled anesthesia pump, or even consultation with the pain service, facilitates any rehabilitation steps.

No matter what injury we discuss and the procedures accomplished to make the patient whole, the patient has to be motivated and compliant. The lack of both can impede healing, which prolongs recovery. We can pick and choose elective surgical cases if suspicions exist that the patient may be noncompliant. Patients with trauma afford us no such luxury.

Discharge planning can begin as early as admission. A social worker could inquire whether the patient needs a subacute or rehabilitation facility. Arrangements are made depending on patient preference, insurance coverage, and bed availability. If the patient is injured while working, the insurance carrier may have their own case worker responsible for placement. Home health care can also be arranged if a formal facility is considered to be too extensive.

Sometimes, a person sustains foot and ankle trauma while traveling in your area. Follow-up visits are in their home state. For continuity of care, the foot and ankle surgeon should locate a colleague in that area, discuss the case, and forward pertinent studies. The receiving physician should then forward periodic reports to the referring physician.

The various fractures, sprains, or strains have specific parameters for when rehabilitation in the form of physical therapy should begin.[4] Not all require a formal physical therapy consultation. Some may suffice with simple at-home active and passive exercises. Others need many sessions of structured physical therapy. One type of fracture does not equate to an automatic physical therapy. For example, however many times ankle fractures are fixated, everything else being equal, 1 patient has a decreased range of motion needing therapy and another's range of motion is equal to the contralateral side (**Fig. 1**). The latter neither receives nor needs any physical therapy.

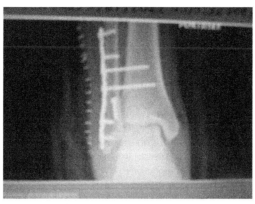

Fig. 1. Open reduction internal fixation of ankle fracture. Patient had a normal range of ankle motion postoperatively and did not require physical therapy.

Egol and colleagues[5] looked at ankle fractures postoperatively. One group was immobilized in a cast, the other in a conventional brace. Physical therapy in the former was started after cast removal; in the latter, almost immediately. Those braced had better outcome scores and returned to work earlier. Any therapy, but especially weight bearing, started too early, may complicate fracture healing.

A compliant patient could have the removable cast boot applied at week 2 and removed periodically to initially begin gentle range of motion exercises. Sensing that a patient may be noncompliant, the duration of immobilization in a short leg cast may be longer versus a removable cast boot. A quick transition in the noncompliant patient may jeopardize the results.

Typically, physical therapy is prescribed for 4 to 6 weeks, 3 times per week. The facility has to be part of the patient's insurance coverage and may require preauthorization. Workman's compensation cases may direct the patient to a particular physical therapy practice. The foot and ankle surgeon should be familiar with the place of therapy. Frequent updates are forwarded to the physician. At the end of the first prescription of 4 to 6 weeks, the patient is seen to determine if another period should be ordered. Some improvement in strength, lessened edema, less pain, and increased range of motion point to the benefits of physical therapy. The key is to know when additional physical therapy is not warranted either because of achievement of the goals or because maximum benefit has been reached. In some instances, the therapist cannot do more and the goals are not met.

From a practical standpoint, 2 periods of physical therapy, whether at 8 or 12 weeks, seem to be adequate to reach goals. An insurance carrier with a work injury may dictate where and how much physical therapy is warranted. However, physical therapy may have to be continuously renewed after multiple surgeries; for example, after open reduction internal fixation (ORIF) of an ankle fracture, and then, after hardware removal. An appeal can be made to the insurance carrier if the physician believes that physical therapy was discontinued too soon.

Patients who complain of leaving therapy in pain are not being treated correctly. The mantra "no pain, no gain" has lost favor when rehabilitating an injury. However, the physician has to determine if the patient wants to be coddled too much, whether out of fear of pain, or has a motive not to get well too rapidly.

Specific modalities are ordered when writing the physical therapy prescription. The prescription lists the diagnosis, duration of physical therapy in weeks, the number of

Wallace

sessions per week, and the modalities. Adding "ad lib" is not specific enough and gives the therapist too much latitude.

An emphasis on patient compliance is sought both by the foot and ankle surgeon and by the therapist. Communication between both has to be open and frank. A malingering patient is identified at the earliest point.

The doctor-patient relationship in a traumatic situation is a quick introduction, without the luxury of being given recommendations from other patients, inquiring about the physician, and choosing to make an appointment. The first meeting is under duress and unpleasant circumstances: the patient just had a traumatic foot and ankle event and the physician just happened to be on call that day. That first impression can have a major impact on the relationship. The relationship can be quickly dissolved if the insurance is an issue. Some plans allow the emergent care, including surgery and possibly, 1 postoperative visit. Then, the patient is taken from the physician, unless appealed, to follow up at a participating provider or one sanctioned by the insurance carrier.

As rehabilitation progresses, the foot and ankle surgeon has the responsibility to chart accurately. Unique to the injured foot and ankle, if unilateral, is the ability to compare and contrast the affected side with the contralateral one. An experiment is taking place using the injured side versus a control, the contralateral uninjured side. Findings on both sides are reported.

A few questions to keep in mind as physical therapy is performed:

1. Why is the edema not decreasing?
2. Why has the range of motion not improved?
3. Is the hardware causing pain? Williams and colleagues[6] reported a 91% satisfaction rate after implant removal. Fixation in this region may have less soft tissue coverage with the demands of weight bearing.
4. Is this a workman's compensation case?
5. Has the patient developed a drug dependency?
6. Has the patient reached maximum medical improvement (MMI) and the results are final?
7. Would a second opinion help?
8. Could the physical therapy be improved either by adding modalities or changing the facility?
9. Is the patient ready for a custom shoe/brace?
10. Is the injured part nonsalvageable and better managed with an amputation?
11. Is the physical therapist providing accurate documentation matching your findings?
12. Did you call for an update?

Depression after a traumatic event can occur and impede progress. It is more problematic in those in whom rehabilitation is perceived to be too slow, a job may be lost, or the final outcome is one of pain and dysfunction. A referral to a behavior specialist may be in order.

PAIN

Ever since pain became the fifth vital sign, both patient and physician have become aware of its presence. The foot and ankle surgeon wants to mitigate the pain as much as possible, but without causing dependency. The patient naturally does not want to experience pain and can be demanding in their requests. Pain is purely subjective and, with the absence of any clinical signs, the physician has to take the patient's word for it.

Pain control begins intraoperatively and while the patient is hospitalized. The use of multimodal analgesic therapy, as a therapeutic benefit, can also reduce hospital stay.[7]

Part of the team should include a pain specialist. They are invaluable, especially in 5 scenarios:

1. The patient with a complex foot and ankle trauma (eg, a crush injury)
2. The patient not responding to analgesics
3. The patient suspected of being, or who is, drug dependent
4. The patient who needs to have complex regional pain syndrome (CRPS) ruled in or out; if diagnosed, then rapid treatment is initiated
5. The patient on methadone and previous history of dependency

Using this list, the pain specialist even becomes a second opinion. Their findings are included in the patient's chart.

After trauma, there are 3 issues that have to be developed further. The first is Charcot arthropathy developing on the injured side in a susceptible patient. However, the contralateral lower extremity has to be examined regularly. Diabetics, as part of the initial traumatic physical examination, are checked for neuropathy. Some may not know that they are diabetic or neuropathic. Fixation is increased, and the duration for bone healing is at least double those without neuropathy. Complications are greater in those with complicated diabetes than in those with neurologic or vascular issues.[8]

Second, the patient is asked about calf pain and examined to determine if a deep vein thrombophlebitis (DVT) is present. This examination should be performed during every visit. Any suspicion should warrant further testing. It is not the intent of this article to discuss who requires DVT prophylaxis.

Third, those with either subtle or easily recognizable signs of CRPS should be granted a pain consultation. Any suspicion of CRPS warrants an immediate pain referral. The earlier the diagnosis and treatment, the greater the chance of relief.[9]

These issues are in addition to those complications encountered more frequently: a postoperative infection, wound healing events, osseous problems, and induration. By no means is this list all inclusive.

The patient with trauma may have a plethora of comorbidities and be on a multitude of medications. Good medical management is therefore necessary. These factors are taken into consideration in the entire perioperative period.

All of these issues show the importance of index of suspicion in medical practice. Those 3 words may be the most cogent used on a daily basis.[10] Suspicion leads to action rather than delay. These 3 entities have to be identified quickly and acted on.

FOOT AND ANKLE TRAUMA AT WORK

A subset of foot and ankle trauma with its own set of verbiage and protocols is the patient who is injured at work. Overall, workplace injuries comprise 20% of all injuries. Foot and ankle traumas are 10% of those injuries.[11]

Initially, nothing is different when treating the injury. A crush injury does not change its presentation or treatment just because it was the result of an accident at work. What follows is what can make such an injury challenging.

Part of the history in these patients is their occupation and what they were doing at the time of injury. Documentation of these items is included in the chart.[12] Occupational history is also important as a baseline for whether the injured patient can return to their occupation. In addition, occupational therapy may be required.[13]

Usually, the insurance carrier wants a copy of the report of each visit almost immediately after the visit. The requests are made through an assigned case manager. The entries are scrutinized. Questions may be asked regarding a particular finding or treatment selection. Also, there are the obvious questions: "When can the patient return to work?" "At full duty?" "When can the patient return to light duty?" In some industries, no light duty is available.

Surprisingly, the patient may not have personal health insurance. However, the employer is required to have disability insurance for the employees. This insurance is not in place if the worker is not on the books.

CASE STUDY

Another aspect of an injury at work is shown by the following case study.

A 30-year-old laborer was operating a piece of machinery. His left foot became lodged in the conveyor belt. The dead man's switch was not in reach. His frantic yells alerted a coworker, who stopped the machine and pulled him free. Two hours later he was evaluated. Radiographs depicted closed nondisplaced second, third, and fourth metatarsal fractures (**Fig. 2**). Because of the mechanism of injury, metatarsal fractures, pain out of proportion, pain with passive and active motion, paresthesias, and marked edema, a compartment syndrome was suspected. The pressure in the first interspace was 41 mm Hg and the medial 49 mm Hg. The patient had emergent fasciotomies, with large hematomas evacuated from the 3 fasciotomy incisions. Three days later, the medial calcaneal incision was closed primarily and the 2 dorsal ones closed with split-thickness skin grafts. The patient was discharged the next day and followed in the clinic in 1 week.

During the initial postoperative visit, there were no signs of infection, a marked decrease in edema, with almost no pain. The skin grafts were charted at almost 100% take. The areas were redressed, the posterior splint reapplied, and an appointment was made to return in 1 week. The patient never showed. The insurance carrier was contacted and said that the rest of the care would be supplied by their doctor.

This case history is not by any means a solitary case. Often, 1 postoperative visit is granted, and then, the patient moves to another physician, who does not have to be of a similar specialty.

Likewise, if the injured worker has insurance X, and the doctor/facility does not take insurance X, the patient is granted 1 postoperative visit. If there are no out-of-network benefits, then, the patient is lost. One may request updates, but they occur rarely.

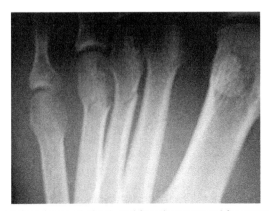

Fig. 2. Nondisplaced closed second, third, and fourth metatarsal fractures after the foot was caught in a conveyor belt.

The Occupational Safety and Health Administration (OSHA) may be brought in to investigate the location of the dead man's switch in relation to the worker and how easily it could be activated. If OSHA found a violation, the employer could be fined and the machine revamped.

WORKMAN'S COMPENSATION

The following is used to show a workman's compensation case that one treats from the beginning to the end.

A 25-year-old warehouse worker was hit by a Hi Lo and sustained a closed trimalleolar ankle fracture necessitating ORIF (**Figs. 3** and **4**). Discharge was the day after surgery.

On the second postoperative visit and for most of the subsequent visits, the assigned case worker from the insurance company accompanied the patient. At a rate of every other visit, a picture of the site was taken. A brief form at each visit was filled out listing the findings, next appointment, and estimated return to work date. The next day, the case worker called for a copy of the notes. Physical therapy was approved but had to be at a site authorized by the carrier.

It is difficult to estimate a date for return to work. In this case, the worker was in a warehouse on his feet the entire time. Return in 3, 4, or 6 months? Some employers are able to accommodate the worker doing a job different from their normal occupation (eg, sitting at a desk). Others want to know when the employee can return for light duty at their same occupation, at how many hours per day, and for how many weeks. Some have no light duty; it is all or nothing (**Box 1**). Any dates supplied for a return to work in any capacity are estimates.

An example is to return to light duty at the 4-month mark, 4 hours per day, for 1 month. Without difficulties after this strategy, the patient would then be cleared to return to full duty. Even although cleared for return, some patients may not be able to return after a trial period and request permanent disability. Others may be easier to identify that a return to their occupation is impossible.

WORKER'S COMPENSATION BENEFITS

The injured worker receives benefits while not working, although states vary with rules and regulations regarding benefits permitted during a specific period. This situation, then, would be considered temporary disability.

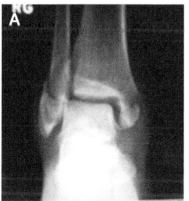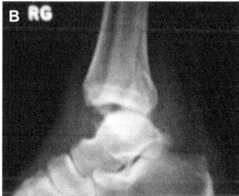

Fig. 3. Trimalleolar ankle fracture. (*A*) Anteroposterior view. (*B*) Lateral view.

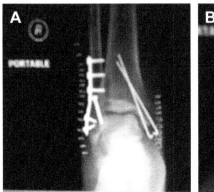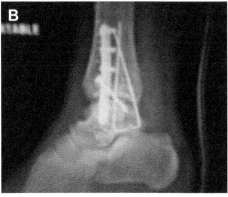

Fig. 4. ORIF of trimalleolar ankle fracture. (*A*) Anteroposterior view. (*B*) Lateral view.

Box 1
An example of an insurance form, which is completed at every visit

Please address the following at this appointment:

Work Related?   Yes   No (Please explain)

Exam / Findings (CPT codes) Confirm diagnosis_____

Recommendations & Treatment Plan / PT – frequency, modalities, duration. Please include RX (Script) if applicable. Also, send all medical including Operative Report.

☐ NO WORK _____
☐ ESTIMATE RETURN _____
☐ MAXIMUM MEDICAL IMPROVEMENT (MMI) DATE: _____
☐ RETURN TO WORK WITHOUT RESTRICTIONS AS OF DATE: _____
☐ RETURN TO WORK WITH FOLLOWING RESTRICTIONS AS OF: _____

    ☐ Sedentary work only
    ☐ No work requiring repetitive or prolonged kneeling, squatting, or climbing
    ☐ No lifting over   10   25   50   75   100 lbs
    ☐ No work requiring use of arms above shoulder level
    ☐ No operating of mobile equipment
    ☐ No work requiring repetitive or prolonged bending or stooping
    ☐ No work requiring prolonged walking and/or standing

Additional Comments: _____

Next Appointment is scheduled for: _____

PHYSICIAN SIGNATURE_____

There is a determination that the patient has reached MMI. MMI is reached when there is no further improvement and the patient has stabilized. The physical therapist may declare from their own standpoint that MMI has been obtained.

MMI has to be realistic from both the patient's and physician's standpoint. Malingering has to be considered. MMI does not imply that the patient is now at preinjury levels but does suggest that based on the injury, all treatments, including consultations, have come to an end point with what exists. The patient may not be agreeable with the MMI designation. There is always the specter of fraud and abuse. At this juncture, an independent medical examiner (IME) may be requested by the insurance carrier. The IME determines whether there is a partial or total disability. Not only does this decision affect work status but it sets the stage for any monetary compensation for the injury over the worker's projected career and earning potential.

The IME can perform a functional capacity evaluation (FCE) looking at the patient's ability to perform tasks related to their job.[14] The American Medical Association *Guides to the Evaluation of Permanent Improvement, Sixth Edition* rates impairment. The guides are useful in determining an injury and clinical findings percentage (if not 100%) of disability (**Box 2**).

The patient may not be satisfied with the result. Legal representation may be sought to adjudicate a better settlement. A lawyer, usually one specializing in compensation cases, may be brought in to sue the employer for an unsafe work environment, the patient's being injured on the job, and for a larger monetary settlement. Treatment notes are admissible. The foot and ankle surgeon may be asked to testify as the treating physician. The amount of acrimony between the parties may determine if a settlement can be reached without appearing in court.

Besides disability forms, ancillary forms to be completed may include a handicap placard for a car, a change or cancellation of gym membership, and deferment of financial obligations.

THE DIFFERENCE IF INJURED ON THE JOB

Kunkel and Miller[13] determined that the sooner the patient was able to return to work, the better. Yet, when studies on injuries are conducted and published, the worker's compensation cases are either not included in the results or their results are poor compared with those without a work injury.[5,15,16]

Seland and colleagues[17] determined that temporary disability was increased in older workers, women, construction workers, and those falling from a height. Duration of time off could be modified by the following: adequacy of treatment, contact with

---

Box 2
Terms for the injured worker

1. Case worker

2. Worker's compensation benefits

3. MMI

4. Temporary disability

5. Permanent disability

6. IME

7. FCE

work, perceived disability, coping mechanisms, workplace accommodations, the nature of work, fear of nonrecovery, and patient expectations. Intuitively, there seems to be a triumverate operating with all work-related cases: the patient, physician, and employer. The lines of communication and thorough expectations have to be made known to all. A workplace injury can almost do the opposite, creating an adversarial relationship between the patient and employer. The physician is in the middle, with allegiance, naturally, to the patient.

Mason and colleagues[18] compared workplace versus nonworkplace injuries. Those with the former usually had less severe injuries, were older, married, and more likely to partake in litigation. They blamed either another worker or equipment. Some may get better quickly on settlement.

Even something as simple as a toe amputation can lead to temporary disability of a mean of 4 months.[19] In the Canadian study, this procedure was not an insignificant economic episode.

A CASE STUDY

A patient fell on an icy sidewalk and sustained a trimalleolar ankle fracture. Two weeks after ORIF, there was an infection. Subsequently, she needed a free flap. She had worked for her company for more than 20 years. Because of her prolonged absence of 9 months, her employment was terminated. A lawyer was brought in to sue the property owner where the fall occurred. Lost wages and future earnings are part of the litigation.

SUMMARY

Patients with foot and ankle trauma are a unique cohort. These patients arrive with a problem that needs attention. Age and comorbidities may have precluded them from having elective bunion surgery, for example, but because of circumstances, they need treatment. Recovery could be long and arduous, and rehabilitation is often necessary. Those injured at work are accompanied with all the paperwork and protocols such an injury entails. All parties have to be satisfied in a work-related injury: the physician, worker, employer, and the insurer.

REFERENCES

1. Sanders R, Fortin P, DiPisquale T, et al. Operative treatment in 120 displaced intraarticular calcaneal fractures: results using a prognostic computed tomography scan classification. Clin Orthop 1993;290:87–95.
2. Colaizzi T. Pedorthic considerations in the management of the injured worker. Foot Ankle Clin 2002;7:403–8.
3. Ruedi T, Buckley RE, Moran CG. AO philosophy and evolution. In: Ruedi T, Buckley RE, Moran CG, editors. AO principles of fracture management. New York: Thieme; 2007. p. 1–7.
4. Ryf CR, Arraf J. Postoperative management: general considerations. In: Ruedi T, Buckley RE, Moran CG, editors. AO principles of fracture management. New York: Thieme; 2007. p. 447–67.
5. Egol KA, Dolan R, Koval KJ. Functional outcome of surgery for fractures of the ankle. J Bone Joint Surg Br 2000;3:246–9.
6. Williams AA, Witten DM, Duester R, et al. The benefits of implant removal from the foot and ankle. J Bone Joint Surg Am 2012;94:1316–20.

7. Michelson JD, Addante RA, Charlson MD. Multimodal analgesia therapy reduces length of hospitalization in patients undergoing fusions of the ankle and hind foot. Foot Ankle Int 2013;34:1526–34.
8. Wukich DK, Joseph A, Ryan M, et al. Outcomes of ankle fractures in patients with uncomplicated versus complicated diabetes. Foot Ankle Int 2011;32:120–30.
9. Lee KJ, Kirchner JS. Complex regional pain syndrome and chronic pain management in the lower extremity. Foot Ankle Clin 2002;7:409–19.
10. Groopman J. How doctors think. Boston: Houghton Mifflin; 2007.
11. Conti SF, Silverman L. Epidemiology of foot and ankle injuries in the workplace. Foot Ankle Clin 2007;7:273–90.
12. Vanichkachorn G, Roy BA, Lopez R, et al. Evaluation and treatment of the acutely injured worker. Am Fam Physician 2014;89:17–24.
13. Kunkel M, Miller SD. Return to work after foot and ankle injury. Foot Ankle Clin 2002;7:421–8.
14. Lechner DE. The role of functional capacity evaluation in management of foot and ankle dysfunction. Foot Ankle Clin 2002;7:449–76.
15. Myerson MS, McGarvey WC, Henderson MR, et al. Morbidity after crush injuries to the foot. J Orthop Trauma 1994;8:343–9.
16. Calder JDF, Whitehouse SL, Saxby TS. Results of isolated Lisfranc injuries and the effect of compensation claims. J Bone Joint Surg Br 2004;86:527–30.
17. Seland K, Cherry N, Beach J. A study of factors influencing return to work after wrist or ankle fractures. Am J Ind Med 2006;49:197–203.
18. Mason S, Wardrope TG, Turpin G, et al. Outcomes after injury: a comparison of workplace and nonworkplace injuries. J Trauma 2002;53:98–103.
19. Hebert JS, Ashworth NL. Predictors of return to work following traumatic work-related lower extremity amputations. Disabil Rehabil 2006;28:613–8.

Supramalleolar Osteotomy and Ankle Arthrodiastasis for Juvenile Posttraumatic Ankle Arthritis

John J. Stapleton, DPM[a,b,*], Thomas Zgonis, DPM[c]

KEYWORDS

- Internal fixation • External fixation • Ankle deformity • Arthrodiastasis
- Supramalleolar osteotomy • Posttraumatic arthritis

KEY POINTS

- In the juvenile patient, posttraumatic ankle arthritis with an associated lower extremity deformity presents a surgical dilemma to the treating physician.
- Combined supramalleolar osteotomy and ankle arthrodiastasis can provide a viable surgical option in the younger population.
- Ankle joint–sparing procedures can be combined with lower extremity deformity correction.

Juvenile patients with posttraumatic arthritis and deformity of the ankle joint can present a surgical challenge to the treating physician. Even though numerous surgical procedures have been described for the adult population, ankle arthroplasty or arthrodesis may not be as feasible for the juvenile patient. Joint-sparing procedures consist of, but are not limited to, ankle arthroscopy with synovectomy, realignment supramalleolar osteotomy, ankle arthrodiastasis, and/or a combination of these procedures. This article discusses a combined supramalleolar osteotomy and ankle arthrodiastasis in a juvenile patient with symptomatic end-stage posttraumatic ankle arthritis and valgus deformity.

CASE REPORT

A 16 year old girl presented with symptomatic posttraumatic ankle arthritis after she had sustained an open ankle fracture dislocation at the age of 15 years, which was

[a] Foot and Ankle Surgery, VSAS Orthopaedics, Lehigh Valley Hospital, 1250 South Cedar Crest Boulevard, Suite #110, Allentown, PA 18103, USA; [b] Penn State College of Medicine, 500 University Drive, Hershey, PA 17033, USA; [c] Division of Podiatric Medicine and Surgery, Department of Orthopaedic Surgery, University of Texas Health Science Center San Antonio, 7703 Floyd Curl Drive, MSC 7776, San Antonio, TX 78229, USA
* Corresponding author. VSAS Orthopaedics, 1250 South Cedar Crest Boulevard, Suite 110, Allentown, PA.
E-mail address: jostaple@hotmail.com

Clin Podiatr Med Surg 31 (2014) 597–601
http://dx.doi.org/10.1016/j.cpm.2014.08.001
0891-8422/14/$ – see front matter © 2014 Elsevier Inc. All rights reserved.

treated with a spanning external fixator and delayed osteosynthesis of the medial malleolus and placement of syndesmotic screws. The syndesmotic screws were removed at approximately 3 months after surgery. The patient reported severe pain with prolonged standing and ambulation despite conservative treatment options that consisted of physical therapy modalities, ankle foot orthosis, and gait assistive devices. On physical examination, the neurovascular status was intact with healed incisions over the medial malleolus and distal fibula and without any clinical signs of infection. On standing, a significant valgus deformity at the ankle was evident and the patient displayed a compensatory recurvatum of the knee to obtain a plantigrade foot. The patient ambulated with an antalgic gait that displayed significant external rotation at the hip. Dorsiflexion of the ankle was significantly limited and an anterior bone block impingement was evident. The ankle joint displayed a joint effusion and crepitation with attempted range of motion. Standing radiographs of the ankle and hindfoot alignment radiographs revealed an end-stage posttraumatic osteoarthritis with widening of the ankle mortise, valgus, and procurvatum deformity of the ankle as a result of a malunited fibula fracture. Treatment options discussed with the patient and family consisted of an ankle arthrodesis versus a realignment osteotomy with ankle arthrodiastasis.

SURGICAL TECHNIQUE

After the retained hardware was removed through minimal incisions directly over the medial malleolus, a 4-cm incision was made over the anterior aspect of the distal metaphysis of the tibia. The neurovascular bundle and extensor tendons were mobilized after the extensor retinaculum was incised. At this point, a half pin was placed under C-arm fluoroscopy from anterior to posterior directly in the center of the planned focal dome osteotomy. A Rancho Cube was then loosely attached to the half pin creating a guide for the focal dome osteotomy.[1] Multiple drill holes were placed with a 3.2-mm drill bit to begin and create the curvature for the focal dome osteotomy. The focal dome osteotomy was then completed with a curved osteotome, preserving the surrounding periosteum. At this point, the distal fibula was exposed and a fibula osteotomy performed with a straight osteotome under C-arm fluoroscopic guidance. The fibula osteotomy was placed in alignment with the focal dome osteotomy of the tibia to allow deformity correction. After mobilization of the osteotomy, the valgus deformity of the ankle was corrected along with placing the ankle in 5° to 7° of recurvatum with slight posterior translation to correct for the procurvatum deformity. The osteotomy of the tibia was then fixated with a 6.5-mm cannulated screw placed from the medial malleolus across the osteotomy, and the fibula was then fixated with a one-third tubular plate. A multiplane circular external fixator that consisted of 2 tibia rings (tibia block) and a foot plate was used to perform the ankle arthrodiastasis. The previously placed half pin was secured to the distal tibia ring. The tibia block was then secured to the leg with tensioned smooth wires placed in the lower extremity anatomic safe zones. The foot was then secured to the foot plate with opposing olive wires in the calcaneus and multiple smooth wires placed across the midfoot and forefoot. Hinges were then placed at the level of the ankle joint axis to allow range of motion after surgery. The ankle was then distracted approximately 7 mm under C-arm fluoroscopic guidance.

After surgery, the patient was non–weight bearing for 2 weeks until complete wound healing had occurred. The patient was then permitted to partial weight-bearing status with crutches with physical therapy initiation for supervised ankle joint range of motion. The external fixation device allowed the physical therapist to disconnect the

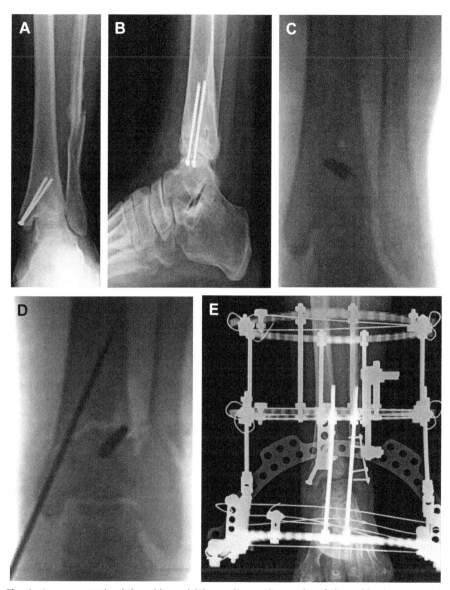

Fig. 1. Anteroposterior (*A*) and lateral (*B*) standing radiographs of the ankle showing end-stage posttraumatic ankle arthritis and deformity in a juvenile patient. Note the valgus tilt of the talus, widening of the medial clear space, shortening and malunion of the fibula, and procurvatum deformity. Intraoperative C-arm fluoroscopic images (*C, D*) showing placement of the half pin in the center of the planned focal dome osteotomy followed by the focal dome osteotomy created initially with drill holes and completed with an osteotome. Note the correction of the ankle mortise. Postoperative anteroposterior (*E*) and lateral (*F*) radiographs of the ankle and lower extremity showing simultaneous ankle arthrodiastasis with a multiplane circular external fixator. The ankle joint was distracted 7 mm and hinges were placed at the level of the ankle joint axis to permit range of motion while the joint was distracted. Final anteroposterior (*G*) and lateral (*H*) weight-bearing radiographs at 22 months after surgery showing realignment of the ankle mortise, healed supramalleolar osteotomy, and evidence of posttraumatic ankle arthritis.

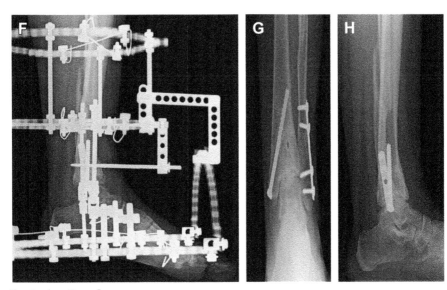

Fig. 1. (continued)

attachment that secured the foot plate to the distal tibia ring and perform range of motion through the hinges that were placed. The external fixator was removed at 4 months after surgery and the patient used a removable fracture boot for an additional 4 weeks before progressing to regular shoe gear. Physical therapy continued for 2 months after surgery to improve range of motion, lower extremity strength, and proprioception.

At 6 months after surgery, radiographs revealed well-healed osteotomies and the patient noticed improved range of motion and ambulation but persistent pain that limited her activities. At 1 year after surgery, the patient reported only intermittent minor discomfort and a normal gait pattern, whereas at 22 months after surgery the patient was pleased with her functional outcome and pain levels were minimum. At her last follow-up, she revealed improved function, increased range of motion at the ankle joint, and diminished pain despite the radiographic evidence of posttraumatic ankle arthritis (**Fig. 1**).

DISCUSSION

Numerous surgical techniques have been described for posttraumatic ankle arthritis with or without an associated lower extremity deformity in the adult population.[2–7] These surgical procedures include, but are not limited to, ankle exostectomy with joint resurfacing, ankle arthrodiastasis, ankle arthroplasty, ankle arthrodesis, and supramalleolar osteotomy for realignment.

Posttraumatic ankle arthritis in juvenile patients is a surgical challenge because ankle arthroplasty or arthrodesis may not be a feasible option in patients at this age. The rationale for this surgical case was to perform a supramalleolar osteotomy to correct the underlying deformity and to improve ankle range of motion while simultaneously performing an ankle arthrodiastasis to address the symptomatic posttraumatic ankle arthritis. The deformity correction focused on reestablishment of the ankle mortise and realigning the weight-bearing axis through the center of the talus. In addition, the procurvatum of the tibia was corrected with slight recurvatum to allow improved dorsiflexion. To prevent the foot from translating forward, the osteotomy and the center of the ankle joint were translated slightly posteriorly.

SUMMARY

Supramalleolar osteotomy for an ankle deformity correction combined with ankle arthrodiastasis for posttraumatic arthritis is a joint-sparing procedure that may prevent or delay the need for ankle arthrodesis or ankle arthroplasty. Further studies are needed to determine the benefit of this procedure in this patient population.

REFERENCES

1. Mendicino RW, Catanzariti AR, Reeves CL. Percutaneous supramalleolar osteotomy for distal tibial (near articular) ankle deformities. J Am Podiatr Med Assoc 2005;95:72–84.
2. Ugaji S, Watanabe K, Matsubara H, et al. Simultaneous arthrodiastasis and deformity correction for a patient with ankle arthrodiastasis and lower extremity deformity: a case report. Foot Ankle Surg 2014;20:74–8.
3. Sagray BA, Levitt BA, Zgonis T. Ankle arthrodiastasis and interpositional ankle exostectomy. Clin Podiatr Med Surg 2012;29:501–7.
4. Siddiqui NA, Herzenberg JE, Lamm BM. Supramalleolar osteotomy for realignment of the ankle joint. Clin Podiatr Med Surg 2012;29:465–82.
5. Pagenstert GI, Hintermann B, Barg A, et al. Realignment surgery as alternative treatment of varus and valgus ankle osteoarthritis. Clin Orthop Relat Res 2007; 462:156–68.
6. Pagenstert G, Knupp M, Valderrabano V, et al. Realignment surgery for valgus ankle osteoarthritis. Oper Orthop Traumatol 2009;21:77–87.
7. Valderrabano V, Paul J, Monika H, et al. Joint-preserving surgery of valgus ankle osteoarthritis. Foot Ankle Clin 2013;18:481–502.

Index

Note: Page numbers of article titles are in **boldface** type.

Clin Podiatr Med Surg 31 (2014) 603–610
http://dx.doi.org/10.1016/S0891-8422(14)00069-X
0891-8422/14/$ – see front matter © 2014 Elsevier Inc. All rights reserved.

podiatric.theclinics.com

United States Postal Service

Statement of Ownership, Management, and Circulation
(All Periodicals Publications Except Requestor Publications)

1. Publication Title	2. Publication Number	3. Filing Date
Clinics in Podiatric Medicine and Surgery	0 0 0 - 7 0 7	9/14/14

4. Issue Frequency	5. Number of Issues Published Annually	6. Annual Subscription Price
Jan, Apr, Jul, Oct	4	$305.00

7. Complete Mailing Address of Known Office of Publication (Not printer) (Street, city, county, state, and ZIP+4®)

Elsevier Inc.
360 Park Avenue South
New York, NY 10010-1710

Contact Person: Stephen R. Bushing
Telephone (Include area code): 215-239-3688

8. Complete Mailing Address of Headquarters or General Business Office of Publisher (Not printer)

Elsevier Inc., 360 Park Avenue South, New York, NY 10010-1710

9. Full Names and Complete Mailing Addresses of Publisher, Editor, and Managing Editor (Do not leave blank)

Publisher (Name and complete mailing address)

Linda Belfus, Elsevier Inc., 1600 John F. Kennedy Blvd., Suite 1800, Philadelphia, PA 19103-2899

Editor (Name and complete mailing address)

Patrick Manley, Elsevier Inc., 1600 John F. Kennedy Blvd., Suite 1800, Philadelphia, PA 19103-2899

Managing Editor (Name and complete mailing address)

Adrianne Brigido, Elsevier Inc., 1600 John F. Kennedy Blvd., Suite 1800, Philadelphia, PA 19103-2899

10. Owner (Do not leave blank. If the publication is owned by a corporation, give the name and address of the corporation immediately followed by the names and addresses of all stockholders owning or holding 1 percent or more of total amount of stock. If not owned by a corporation, give the names and addresses of the individual owners. If owned by a partnership or other unincorporated firm, give its name and address as well as those of each individual owner. If the publication is published by a nonprofit organization, give its name and address.)

Full Name	Complete Mailing Address
Wholly owned subsidiary of	1600 John F. Kennedy Blvd, Ste. 1800
Reed/Elsevier, US holdings	Philadelphia, PA 19103-2899

11. Known Bondholders, Mortgagees, and Other Security Holders Owning or Holding 1 Percent or More of Total Amount of Bonds, Mortgages, or Other Securities. If none, check box ☐ None

Full Name	Complete Mailing Address
N/A	

12. Tax Status (For completion by nonprofit organizations authorized to mail at nonprofit rates) (Check one)
The purpose, function, and nonprofit status of this organization and the exempt status for federal income tax purposes:
☐ Has Not Changed During Preceding 12 Months
☐ Has Changed During Preceding 12 Months (Publisher must submit explanation of change with this statement)

13. Publication Title	14. Issue Date for Circulation Data Below
Clinics in Podiatric Medicine & Surgery	July 2014

15.	Extent and Nature of Circulation		Average No. Copies Each Issue During Preceding 12 Months	No. Copies of Single Issue Published Nearest to Filing Date
a.	Total Number of Copies (Net press run)		552	533
b. Paid Circulation (By Mail and Outside the Mail)	(1)	Mailed Outside-County Paid Subscriptions Stated on PS Form 3541. (Include paid distribution above nominal rate, advertiser's proof copies, and exchange copies)	358	305
	(2)	Mailed In-County Paid Subscriptions Stated on PS Form 3541 (Include paid distribution above nominal rate, advertiser's proof copies, and exchange copies)		
	(3)	Paid Distribution Outside the Mails Including Sales Through Dealers and Carriers, Street Vendors, Counter Sales, and Other Paid Distribution Outside USPS®	31	35
	(4)	Paid Distribution by Other Classes Mailed Through the USPS (e.g. First-Class Mail®)		
c.	Total Paid Distribution (Sum of 15b (1), (2), (3), and (4))	▶	389	340
d. Free or Nominal Rate Distribution (By Mail and Outside the Mail)	(1)	Free or Nominal Rate Outside-County Copies Included on PS Form 3541	82	105
	(2)	Free or Nominal Rate In-County Copies Included on PS Form 3541		
	(3)	Free or Nominal Rate Copies Mailed at Other Classes Through the USPS (e.g. First-Class Mail)		
	(4)	Free or Nominal Rate Distribution Outside the Mail (Carriers or other means)		
e.	Total Free or Nominal Rate Distribution (Sum of 15d (1), (2), (3) and (4))	▶	82	105
f.	Total Distribution (Sum of 15c and 15e)	▶	471	445
g.	Copies not Distributed (See instructions to publishers #4 (page #3))	▶	81	88
h.	Total (Sum of 15f and g)	▶	552	533
i.	Percent Paid (15c divided by 15f times 100)	▶	82.59%	76.40%

16. Total circulation includes electronic copies. Report circulation on PS Form 3526-X worksheet.

17. Publication of Statement of Ownership
If the publication is a general publication, publication of this statement is required. Will be printed in the October 2014 issue of this publication.

18. Signature and Title of Editor, Publisher, Business Manager, or Owner

Stephen R. Bushing – Inventory Distribution Coordinator

Date: September 14, 2014

I certify that all information furnished on this form is true and complete. I understand that anyone who furnishes false or misleading information on this form or who omits material or information requested on the form may be subject to criminal sanctions (including fines and imprisonment) and/or civil sanctions (including civil penalties).

PS Form 3526, August 2012 (Page 1 of 3 (Instructions Page 3)) PSN 7530-01-000-9931 PRIVACY NOTICE: See our Privacy policy in www.usps.com

PS Form 3526, August 2012 (Page 2 of 3)

Printed and bound by CPI Group (UK) Ltd, Croydon, CR0 4YY

03/10/2024

01040495-0011